D0047440

Oh Sh*t, I Almost Killed You!

A Little Book of Big Things
Nursing School Forgot to Teach You

By Sonja M. Schwartzbach, BSN, RN, CCRN

Oh Shit, I Almost Killed You!
A Little Book of Big Things Nursing School Forgot to Teach You

ISBN 978-0-692-83869-3

Copyright © 2017
Sonja M. Schwartzbach, BSN, RN, CCRN

All rights reserved. No part of this book may be reproduced in any form, except for the inclusion of brief quotations for review, without permission from the author/publisher. Some identifying details have been changed to protect the privacy of individuals.

Although the author and publisher have made every effort to ensure that the information in this book was correct at press time, the author and publisher do not assume and hereby disclaim any liability to any party for any loss, damage, or disruption caused by errors or omissions, whether such errors or omissions result from negligence, accident, or any other cause.

Cover design and production by JM Group™, www.jmmre.com

Author and cover photography by Krissy Breece

Photography ©,www.krissybreecephotography.com

Joseph,

I'm sorry for what I said when I was hungry.
I love you to the stars.

xo,

Big Spoon

FOREWORD

A totally honest book and a must read for every new nurse and seasoned ones too! For the new nurse, get ready as you just won the lottery! Nurse Sonja offers an engaging look at the world of nursing and how to overcome and survive its myriad of challenges. She will give you emotional guidance and mental peace as she relates the world of nursing through your eyes and mind. Sonja will be your inner therapist as you voyage through the chapters of the world of nursing – all wrapped up with a great big bear hug!

For the seasoned nurse, remember what it is like to be new and get a clearer picture of the importance you play in the neophyte nurse's travels through the fast-paced, highly technical hospital setting. Understanding the frustrations and being sensitive to the new nurses' perceptions will help for a smooth transition into one becoming an experienced and competent nurse. Whether you seek inspiration, advice or a laugh on every page – this book is for you with a two-fold purpose. It's a journey from the beginning of your nursing career and every aspect within. Follow the Yellow Brick Road with Sonja! Come along for the ride, she will guide you through your emotional spectrum, for you are not alone!

Secondly, this book offers practical advice for dealing with a range of emotions. Sonja serves as your mental coach, an inner voice along the way. She is your "get you through the day guru;" your mental mentor; and your professional cheerleader! She will inspire you, and offer support and encouragement on your nursing journey!

"Being a Nurse Means"

You will never be bored.
You will always be frustrated.
You will be surrounded by challenges.
So much to do and so little time.
You will carry immense responsibility
and very little authority.
You will step into people's lives
and you will make a difference.
Some will bless you.
Some will curse you.
You will see people at their worst –
and at their best.
You will never cease to be amazed
at people's capacity for
love, courage, and endurance.
You will see life begin – and end.
You will experience resounding triumphs
and devastating failures.
You will cry a lot.
You will laugh a lot.
You will know what it is to be human
and to be humane.
Melodie Chenevert, RN

I can't wait for you to read this inspiring book
as it is an asset to professionals
stepping foot into a new environment!

Good luck to you!
Much success in your new life as a nurse!

Laura Gasparis Vonfrolio RN, PhD

ACKNOWLEDGEMENTS

This is the very last piece of my book, and the part where I immediately start to panic. While I want to express gratitude to every single person in my life who has touched me in some way (figuratively, I think), I understand one very crucial detail: this book isn't f*cking *War and Peace*. It's not some work of literary genius, nor is it going to ever revolutionize mankind. BUT, it is, indeed, my baby – and while your first child may cause you the most grief, it is also usually your favorite. This nursey non-fiction lovechild could never have been conceived without some incredibly important people in my life. First and foremost, I thank Dr. Laura Gasparis Vonfrolio for being my nursing Fairy Godmother and turning my manuscript into reality. I extend gratitude to Mr. Jack Berens and JM Group™ team for web design and creative expertise; Mrs. Krissy Breece for making photo magic despite frigid temperatures; Mr. Daniel Boudwin, Esq. for his legal know-how; and Ms. Sehr Thadhani, marketing genius extraordinaire.

On a more personal front, I would never have had the courage to press forward throughout brain farts and writer's blocks without the support of my cheerleading parents and in-laws; my brilliant sisters; my supportive colleagues; and my amazing friends. I have been blessed to give, learn, and grow with a deliciously dysfunctional group of clinical dynamos, without whom I could never evolve into the potty-mouthed ICU nurse that I am today. Angela, Bonnie, Claire: I owe you each a cut. And as for my husband? He is the ground while I live with my head in the clouds. I thank him for the countless loads of laundry and encouraging forehead kisses that landed just as I needed them.

Finally: to my readers, I thank you from the very bottom of my heart. Every note, comment, and email inspired me to bring this idea to reality. I cannot thank you enough for validating what I do…what *we* do…even when – especially if – it's off the beaten path.

xo

Sonja

The Ten New Nurse Commandments

1) Thou shalt not forget to drinketh coffee before your shift, pee during your shift, and find a way to relax after your shift.

2) Thou shalt document it, for it has been done.

3) Thou shalt honor thy medications and the six rights of administration. (*Six? Hold on, there are SIX rights now? Was five not enough?! Whatever. Right drug. Right dose. Right route. Right time. Right patient. Right documentation – see commandment two above*).

4) Thou shalt compress hard and compress fast; push the Epi every three to five minutes; and only shocketh a shockable rhythm.

5) Thou shalt give thy Colace, for impaction is a sin.

6) Thou shalt pay homage to the holy nursing trinity: Ativan, Haldol, and Propofol.

7) Thou shalt sleep between shifts, even if only for a few hours.

8) Thou shalt wash thy hands before you enter, after you exit, and between patient care.

9) Thou shalt scrub thy hub.

10) Thou shalt treat nurses and colleagues the way you want to be treated, even when others speaketh like assholes.

PART I

OH SHIT! I'M A NURSE NOW!
Corporate Sucker to Candy Striper

I was totally freaking clueless. I sat on a cold NJ Transit train, stalled once again between Newark and Secaucus, feeling sorry for myself and the cards life had dealt. My corporate job sucked, and every day that I left the office I felt a piece of my twenty-three year old soul grow further disengaged. After a particularly bad day – one that, in hindsight, was more likely contrived of a marketing disaster and a Blackberry emergency than anything that was actually meaningful – I pulled out a scrap of paper and started to doodle my thoughts. I'd made a habit of writing to work through whatever I was thinking. From to-do lists to existential musings, I have always solved my problems by throwing them onto a notepad or a cocktail napkin to see what sticks.

So I sat there in uncomfortable silence, crammed between two ornery commuters during the height of rush hour, and allowed my mind to explore my options. Though my original plan had been to work for my media firm and attend law school, I quickly became distressed in finding this plan totally sucked – at least for me, it did. I had already become bored, felt shallow, and was itching to change directions in order to achieve something that could affect the greater good. I was far too social to win a Nobel Prize in astronomy or physics, and I liked food too much and cursed too often to go the Gandhi route. What could I do? Where could I go? How could I serve humanity, feed my soul, and – oh by the way – pay my bills while doing it?

Then it hit me! It was a lightening bulb above the head, Eureka in the bathtub kind of moment: it came speeding at me like a freight train, which, ironically, was the reason my train wasn't moving. I asked myself what I was looking for in a career, and I scribbled down three hopes in my profession: to give, to learn, and to grow. *A nurse! I had to become a nurse! Why didn't I consider nursing before? How come I never felt compelled to pursue such a noble, highly skilled, and overall rewarding profession?*

Well, first of all, I had no idea what nurses actually did. As an eighteen-year-old kid, if you would have told me that I would become a nurse some day I would look at you like you have two heads with purple hair. How stupid! Why would I ever become a nurse? I would become a doctor or a lawyer or something equally as prestigious, not some bedpan dumper that passed out medications to confused old people.

My eighteen-year-old self was kind of an asshole, but that's par for the course for basically every eighteen-year-old who is expected to have the presence of mind and awareness of self to actually know what the hell they want to be when they grow up. Truth be told, I'm thirty years old and I still don't have a clue (much to the dismay of my very supportive and patient husband). It wasn't until I met nurses who worked with my mother through her health issues that I even began to recognize their very importance in the grand scheme of the healthcare world. As a matter of fact, nurses are the lubricant that keeps the healthcare motor running smoothly: they manage every bump, hiccup, and issue with tenacity, flexibility, and the ability to think on their feet. Professionally and personally, lubricant is important: don't let anyone tell you otherwise!

The most interesting part about my journey from corporate minion to registered nurse is that I really didn't understand the depth and breadth of body and mind required of nurses in general, and just how much every experience – good and bad – can change you.

My purpose in sharing this background information with you is this: *I know what you're going through.* I get it. Somehow some dean of a university hands you a diploma and you'll embark on a world where you know less than you actually thought you knew before leaving. It's the craziest thing to enter into a profession where the education and clinical components leave you barely prepared enough to place a urinary catheter into a mannequin with almost-sterile technique, yet expects you to walk into the doors of a hospital, guns blazing, ready to take on the complexities of a healthcare system. At the very least, when medical students complete their education, they embark on residency programs that seek to prepare them for years and years, covering a multitude of clinical scenarios they may experience in the future. Sure, they don't know jack at the start of residency, but thanks to relentless effort and countless nurses, they usually make it out alive. As a new graduate, however, my orientation in my first job on a busy, high acuity cardiac transplant unit was six weeks long. Six weeks. Eighteen shifts. And yes, if I was struggling or drowning or cried enough, my boss and nurse educator would have sat me down and soothed and encouraged and maybe even scolded before giving me a few extra weeks to feel reasonably certain that I wasn't going to intentionally walk into a patient room and immediately kill anybody. But that's it. Nursing is sink or swim. Nursing is a whirlwind. Nursing will make you feel like the stupidest and most incompetent professional on the planet, and it's going to ask that you show up the next day and do it all over again. My own experience – though, admittedly, it was a good one – is one that every new nurse can relate to, and seasoned nurses probably remember like it was yesterday.

For our purposes, I will refer to newly minted nurses or nursing students through a variety of terms: newbie; new nurse; new to practice; novice; and maybe even "baby nurse." These terms are not intended to offend or condescend, nor do they imply that you're infantile and require the constant tender loving care of another. Rather, they serve as highly accurate descriptions of how I felt the very first time I had a patient who was actually experiencing real chest pain and not just post-lunch gas. I was a baby nurse: scared, confused, understanding that I had to act but unable to prioritize my prescribed list of functions. Had I existed in a vacuum and been given some time to think about the situation at hand, I could have easily spouted out the textbook treatment for new-onset chest pain: morphine, nitroglycerin, oxygen, blah, blah, blah. But when you have five patients and fifteen family members and three of them are incontinent and one is trying to climb out of bed and the last is a former convicted criminal with a penchant for inviting young blonde nurses into the bathroom for "alone time" – your brain starts to feel like it's been chopped up and pulsed in a blender. My smoothie-brain didn't afford me the insight of taking vitals, checking my orders, obtaining a stat EKG, phoning the cardiologist, and sending appropriate lab specimens. Instead I panicked and searched frantically for my former preceptor, who was ruining my life at that very moment in that she: 1) actually ate lunch; and 2) even left the floor to do it. I could feel the separation anxiety well up within me: despite being "on my own," I still believed the only way I could safely practice patient care was with watchful glances and routine check-ins from my veteran mom-nurse. If I do harbor any abandonment issues in my adult life, it can be traced back directly to this very moment. In a pinch and a panic, I found a nurse not much older than I was to help guide me. This dude had graduated new nurse status: though he only had about one year of nursing experience, compared to my two months, he was the bedside equivalent of Mr. Miyagi. Once I could adequately formulate sentences that described my patient condition, Mr. Miyagi guided me through the traumatic experience. Thankfully, the situation was only horrifying for me and not my patient! We tackled the patient's chest pain stepwise, managing to get it under control with couple of doses of oral medication and some oxygen. Although I was ready to call a code blue on the middle aged man sitting up in bed while speaking on his cell phone and watching the evening news, it turned out that he wasn't going to die, and I hadn't been the one to kill him. The patient was eventually transferred to a step-down unit for some intravenous medication and closer monitoring, and to the best of my knowledge, even survived his epic battle against a novice nurse with barely a clue despite her active license.

When I think back on this experience and so many others – ranging from funny to scary to flat out ridiculous – I understand just how far I've come as a nurse; just how much I've grown in such a short period of time; and the circumstances through which I've accomplished this. I am *by no means* perfect. I don't know everything and I never ever will. But I can prioritize a crisis and I can man-up during a code and I think that I've even saved a life or two while doing it. What compels me to address the newer nurses out there – to help guide them through their infancy in this field – is the fact that I've encountered so many who have nurtured me as a professional, and others who were big bad bullies. Human nature is to protect oneself. Fight or flight. Hunt and gather. Find shelter and safety and overcome whatever is attacking at any given moment. Nursing nature is a lot like human nature, except instead of being attacked by an enemy, it's often members of your own tribe who pummel you. Why nurses are so notorious for treating new members of the profession like shark bait is still beyond me. I can help prepare you mentally and encourage you clinically but what I cannot do is prevent this treatment from happening entirely. There is a sub-culture in the nursing profession that is so ingrained yet painfully ironic that it makes little sense to those on the outside, but younger nurses being tormented by their seniors is nothing new to the profession. On the flip side, there is no shortage of younger/cooler/ holier-than-thou new grads that intend to get a couple years of valuable bedside experience to beef up their resumes before fleeing the scene for greener advanced-practice pastures. Who gets to be the great white and who is the little fish is a flux and fluid role. It's our responsibility to create the shift in paradigm that stops allowing nurse-bloggers to continue making deep-sea analogies in print.

Phew. I digress. Back to my point, which is survival of newbie nurse-dom and progression into the role of a nurturer and leader to another nubile and terrified member of this profession. I've learned so much in the past few years thanks to incredible mentors; fellow new graduate nurse commiserates; and my own hustle to learn and understand what I do to and for my patients. Yet I've also played Monday morning quarterback more times than I can count. If I can help any of you new to the scene feel even the slightest bit more prepared to take on the challenges of working in a hospital (or a nursing home or a rehab facility or in home care or as an educator or in the business world – not all nurses work in hospitals, I absolutely know this!), and maybe even show you that every nurse can tell you about his or her own tips and tricks, mistakes and regrets – well, that would make the organized chaos of working in this field feel a little bit more manageable. Come forth, my friend, as we take a dive deep down to the bottom of these murky waters, in search of some professional treasures! (Did you read that last sentence in a pirate voice? You should definitely go back and re-read it with a Jack Sparrow kind of thing – it makes everything you're about to learn feel far more bad-ass.)

The Hunt: How the Hell Can I Find a Job?

Way back in the day (January 2012), I graduated with my Bachelors of Science in Nursing from a great university with a perfect grade point average and stellar references. But none of this likely would have mattered if I didn't already work as a patient care technician at the hospital where I would eventually become hired as a new graduate. My point is this: everyone keeps talking about this great big nursing shortage that's going to require a butt-load of nurses to fill the retirement gap by 2020, and yet it seems that newly-minted nurses are rarely hired into acute care settings without having connections or some relevant experience. It's the chicken or the egg phenomenon that seems to plague college graduates in every domain, but feels especially pervasive in the setting of nursing: you can apply to one hundred positions and never receive so much as a telephone call in return. I know countless nurses who graduated with phenomenal grades and references that ranged from presidents of hospitals to President Obama, yet took months or even years to be hired into a hospital setting. They quickly realized that any experience is better than nothing at all. Although they did not accept their "dream job" based on their expectations, an initial foray into nursing outside of acute care facilities afforded them the transferrable skill set and financial stability to practice as licensed professionals. The reality is this: if you have plans to graduate from a nursing program; walk into a hospital as a novice nurse;

and be hired immediately into the intensive care unit, labor and delivery, the emergency department, or another "hot ticket" hospital unit – I respectfully advise you to think again. While it is absolutely possible and every circumstance is different, the likely scenario is that you'll be told the position went to someone who possessed some variety of experience first.

I don't want newer nurses out there to feel discouraged or saddened by what I'm telling you. However, I want you to enter your career with realistic expectations and an understanding of how hospitals function. As a brand-spanking-new nurse with a squeaky clean license, you're something of a liability. You require extensive training, monitoring, guidance, and encouragement, and this does not come without cost. The time and financial commitment required in training a new nurse is a large one, and often times staffing, acuity, and personality mix are factors associated with whether a new nurse would fumble or fly.

"But Sonja! Don't you understand?! I'm the Chanel Bag of nursing students! I'm a Bugatti in a class full of bicycles! I deserve this and I want this and I earned this!"

I say with a hug and a smile: absolutely nobody cares what you think you are. The nurse world is a vast and deep ocean, and these days, it takes far more than a fancy resume and a diploma to make a splash. Gone are the days of free cars, sign on bonuses, and the opportunity to cherry pick job preferences: the job market has shifted, and the competition is fierce.

That being said, getting your feet wet with as much clinical experience as possible is a helpful key to your first nursing gig. I know that working during school is sometimes impossible and unrealistic for

10

many students. However, my job as a patient care technician served as invaluable experience and exposure within a high-acuity, high-volume setting. The problem with modern-day BSN programs is that, while you're highly trained in didactic and theory, your actual clinical time seems to come at a premium. There is no way that a traditional BSN program can expose you to everything you need to know as a baby nurse, and this constraint becomes even more evident in Accelerated Nursing programs like my own. There are only so many clinical hours in a day, and there is only so much stuff that you're permitted to see, do, and experience as a student nurse. To me, securing a job as a patient care technician was imperative, not only financially but also for the hands-on experience

If you truly have your heart set on working in a hospital setting after graduation, my advice is to network, beg, borrow, and hustle your way into a hospital in any way that you can before you even take the boards and possess a license. Volunteer work is an excellent way to show face in an institution while helping others. Nursing assistant roles can be hard to come by, however even a per diem or temporary position will help you get your bearings about the workings of a hospital. There are also numerous internship and externship programs for nursing students and new graduates that afford you the chance to mesh with colleagues and throw out your clinical feelers. Volunteering as an EMT is another phenomenal way to expose you to patient care scenarios while gaining clinical expertise. Finally, nurse residency programs are starting to pop up across the country, and thanks to their method of clinical training and academic mentorship, you can use your nursing degree to become a new graduate nurse who has a similar cohort with which to grow. Of course, none of these opportunities come without the dreaded interview…

Shall I Attend my Interview, or Should I Kill Myself?

So you finally get the call: whether it's your first nursing job or your tenth, there's a certain rush of excitement wrapped in nerves smothered in horror when human resources calls to schedule your interview. If you're a newer nurse fresh out of college, this experience can be overwhelming. You've survived midterms and finals; care plans and practicums; you've even passed your freaking boards – and now that you've had a millisecond to breathe, you feel the anxiety of sitting down with one or two or ten nurses and nurse managers and selling yourself as America's Next Top Nurse. How do you prepare? Where do you begin? And how can you separate yourself from every other applicant who might come with more experience, insight, and a better runway catwalk?

The long and short of it is this: be yourself. Your self is good enough. In fact, your self is great! You should be proud of everything you've accomplished and take ownership of how much you've grown since you're first day as a nursing student. So many nurses like me come from non-traditional backgrounds, and the life we led before becoming nurses is equally as important to discuss and describe as our nursing educations. I worked as a waitress and bartender during nursing school in addition to my patient care technician role. The transferrable skills that I possessed from working at a busy college dive bar were equally as valuable – maybe even more so – as my corporate career. Don't short-change yourself and your experiences. When presented in the right light, there is no experience that doesn't count for something.

In keeping with the idea that you remain true to yourself, leave the bullshit at the door. Enhancing your skills and describing your strengths and weaknesses in a positive light are very different from lying on your resume or fabricating experiences. It's the difference between putting a soft Valencia filter on your Instagram selfie, and using a hard Hefe: if you put too much effort into covering up what's really there, eventually, the truth will come out. Human resource managers are trained to sniff out what may not feel authentic. If you lie about what you know or do during your nursing interview, you're only shortchanging yourself. Imagine telling a hiring manager that you're highly skilled at intravenous sticks, and show up on your first day without a clue. Not only is this damaging to your reputation, it's dangerous to your patients. Be forthright about what you feel comfortable doing, and honest in what you don't. An eager learner who can take initiative and exude passion is far more likely to learn and grow than someone who is overly confident bordering on arrogance.

Conversely, being completely intimidated and riddled with anxiety won't help your case, either. The interview process is a scary one, but it's not the end of the world. If you have your mind set on failure, you're probably going to fail. You'll choke. You'll freeze. All because you've fulfilled the catastrophic interview prophesy that you created in your head. Instead, remember this: the human resource managers? They're human. The nurse managers, educators, and staff members? They're people too. Meeting with some physicians? Human. And while I cannot confirm with

14

100% certainty that some aren't robots due to their monotone personality and repetitious nature, I can say that it's highly unlikely you're going to be meeting with actual Artificial Intelligence. Whether you're twenty years old or a baby boomer and beyond, you're an adult with skills, brains, and the capacity to take any challenge to task. If you maintain this mindset – one of passion coupled with quiet confidence – you'll nail your first interview and every one that follows.

What Are They Going to Ask Me, and How Do I Respond?

I've had many new nurses and nursing students come to me for advice regarding the hospital interview process, and just what to expect from the interviewers. I think it's safe to assume that the dreaded, "So, tell me about yourself," will be first on the docket in one form or another. Besides looking professional and showing up on time (early is on time, and on time is late – write that on a post it and remember it well), understanding that your first impression can weigh heavily on the flow of your interview and the direction it can take is key. You should describe your path toward becoming a nurse; your work and clinical experiences; and where you see yourself in the immediate future. But, hold off on describing your entire life's story including what you ate for breakfast. For some of you this will be a fairly straightforward discussion – you perhaps have always known you wanted to become a nurse, and your trajectory would reflect this. Others like myself, however, require a little bit of backstory to guide the interviewer through the winding road that brought you to where you are today. One great tip I received from a nursing school instructor was to use my resume as a guide for my "about me" story. If you hit on points that are contained within your resume, you can beat the interviewer to the punch for a number of questions.

The last piece of advice I can offer is to go beyond the obvious. Absolutely make it a point to review the hospital's website, mission statement, size, services, and departments. If they happen to be a

Magnet® Designated facility, familiarize yourself with the Magnet® website to understand what it means to earn and maintain such a distinction. Chances are you will be asked about nursing sensitive quality indicators in one way or another, so definitely keep up to date with the latest practices and procedures for nurse-driven initiatives, too. Finally, understand that a hospital is a business, and you are an investment. Why should they invest in you? Why should they spend the time, money, and resources to bring you on board? Show them how you can contribute to their practice, and that you won't try to leave them in six months. Even if you know that you want to work for two or three years before applying to school to become a nurse anesthetist, for example, perhaps it's wise to leave that conversation out of the initial interview. The manager might assume that they are being used as a stepping-stone and that you aren't fully invested in the role or the unit itself. When asked about your future goals, be honest – but have some common sense. Would you want to take on an investment so high-risk that tells you it's going to leave you with a raw deal from the onset? Probably not. The line between showing initiative and seeming disinterested is a fine one – again, present yourself in a fashion that would allow for the best outcomes for you and the department that you're entering. "This is what I can give you, and here's what I hope to receive in return." The idea that you should present yourself in a way that represents where you want to be and not necessarily where you are is more than an isolated interview incident: it's a mindset. Practice makes perfect: prepare for the process; run a mock interview with someone close to you; and overdress for the occasion. And whether you were cool as a cucumber or totally bombed, never forget the importance of a graceful exit. Thank your interviewers for their time and consideration, and reiterate the idea with a follow up thank you card or email. It's not just good business sense: it's good manners!

You're Hired! And You Already Want to Quit!

It probably seems like a sick and twisted joke. You've graduated with what is arguably one of the most difficult undergraduate majors possible. You've spent your life savings (and student loans, grants, and scholarships) on enough caffeine to study your way through the nursing boards. You survived the dreaded job interview. And now you're officially going to work as an honest to goodness nurse in a real hospital with real patients and real medications...and real blood...and real traumas...and real cardiac arrests...and real super-bug infections...

Are you sensing a trend here? Just as soon as you accomplish some major feat in the nursing world, there's another challenge that immediately presents itself. While this may seem like an eerily accurate analogy for nursing as a profession, take a deep breath and focus. It's not a sprint, my friend: nursing is a marathon. And until you're sweaty and exhausted and ready to throw up at the end, you're probably not quite at the point where you're going to feel comfortable doing the work you are supposed to be doing. Warning! This is where I remind you that you've already pushed through so very much to get to this place: a position as a registered nurse or licensed practical nurse where you can begin to hone in your skills, refine your craft, and eventually realize that all of the bleary-eyed breakdowns were worth it.

"Shut the hell up, Sonja!"

That's exactly what you're thinking! You're wondering how I could ever remember the night sweats and tremors and feelings of nausea that made you wonder whether you're starting your first day as a nurse or suffering from a case of dysentery. Rest assured: what you have is treatable, and you haven't caught it fording a river while crossing the Oregon Trail. It's a disease that every new nurse contracts, and the only cures are persistence and time. What feels like it may kill you, but hopefully will pass leaving you relatively unharmed, is a case of expert to novice syndrome. You've left nursing school feeling like the top dog! The ace in the hole! You can take a manual blood pressure like a boss. You can auscultate breath sounds like there's no tomorrow. You totally understand the difference between long and short acting insulin. What you've learned in the classroom and what happens in reality? Well, that's what infects you with this horrible affliction.

Right now, there is a baby nurse who is searching online and deep inside for an answer. There is a brand new member of the profession who is questioning his or her calling. There is a newly minted graduate who wonders how school seemed to teach her everything and nothing all at the same time. There is a greener-than-grass new hire that is praying she doesn't kill somebody at work tomorrow, and wonders if she already did yesterday. *Dearest baby nurse*, don't let this scary new world drag you down.

You're going to have moments when you are sitting on a toilet seat for far too long, probably for the first time in your entire shift, and question why you even decided to become a nurse in the first place. **That's okay.**

You're going to have days – many of them – when you plop down in your car after leaving work two hours later than anticipated; and you're going to turn off the radio; and you're going to roll down the windows; and you're going to cry the most painful and ugly cry. **That's okay.**

You're going to have shifts where your head is spinning and your hands are shaking and your brain is thinking faster than your fingers can type. **That's okay.**

You're going to have moments when you clean more bodily fluids in one twelve-hour day than an average person might in a lifetime. You're going to feel that – sometimes – you're the only person on the entire unit, because everyone around you is just as busy as you are. **That's okay.**

You're going to have times when patients yell at you for something you didn't know (that perhaps you should have). They will complain about you to anyone that might listen. They may even become so frustrated with their care that they threaten to leave. And this is going to bother the hell out of you. **That's okay.**

You're gonna listen for twenty minutes and still not hear a damn murmur. **That's okay.**

You're going to have moments when you feel like something "just isn't right" with the patient in your care. You won't have enough experience as a frame of reference for what may be happening, or why. You're probably going to feel helpless in these moments – it's a "tip of the tongue" phenomenon to the highest degree. **That's okay.**

You're going to feel devastated the first time a veteran nurse yells at you – even more so when their reaction is for something nit-picky and non-essential. You're going to mumble something unsavory about them under your breath. **That's okay.**

You're going to call a doctor to clarify an order, and she's going to complain. She's going to want answers, details, vital signs, and a picture of what is happening with your patient, and you're going to word-vomit something that probably makes very little sense to an angry cardiologist at 3:00 am. **That's okay.**

You're going to walk into a room expecting to pass your morning medications and come to find your patient unresponsive. Maybe she's stopped breathing. Perhaps she's lost a pulse. Either way, you're going to bring forward everything you learned in every class, clinical, and scenario – and forget how to do any of it. You're going to scream for help. You're going to look like a deer in headlights. And you're going to wonder, "When the hell am I ever going to be able to be as good as they are?" **That's okay.**

You're going to lose that patient, on an unexpected shift, and in an unexpected way. You're going to think it was your fault. You're going to be riddled with guilt and feel ashamed of how you reacted. You're going to replay that scenario in your head over and over again, and every time wonder why you didn't see it coming. You can't always see it coming. You can't always be the hero. **And that's okay.**

Because someday you will be.

Someday you'll understand the subtleties and nuances that no one can teach you except for time Herself.

Someday you'll be able to balance the full-fledged mountain emergencies with the miniature molehill ones.

Someday you're going to address a patient or family member who is frustrated with a sense of firm yet compassionate care, and will know how to redirect their emotions.

Someday you will call a doctor, and she will thank you for keeping such a close eye on whatever concern you've already handled.

Someday you're going to finally take a lunch break, and it will actually be during lunchtime.

Someday you're going to do chest compressions or inject medications or ventilate a patient, and your paralyzing fear will be replaced by sheer adrenaline.

Someday, somebody is going to die on your watch – but whether it's through blood, sweat, and heroics or a quiet and accepted end – you will have made a difference in the journey of that patient and his or her loved ones.

And while some days you may still feel like a hamster on a wheel, going through the motions just to stay afloat –

Someday you will realize that you are not the one sinking and needing to be saved. Rather, you've grown into a life raft for another baby nurse, insecure and unaware of all of her untapped potential.

Someday you will understand that the nursing profession is perhaps the hardest of them all, but in so many different ways, the most rewarding. And **someday** you will stand up for yourself; stand up for your patients; and stand up to the barriers that impact your highest capacity to care – this day will remind you why you trudged through every tear, scream, and exasperated sigh.

So do not give up, baby nurse: new to the world in which nurses beget nurses; still questioning why nothing ever ends up like the texts books might have said. No matter how bad it feels – no matter how hard it seems – always turn to the nurses who can teach you that one can have a brilliant mind and a beautiful soul; one can be funny when things feel too serious; one can be tough as nails and still be softened by the circumstances; one can make mistakes and still maintain integrity. Stand your ground, baby nurse; ask questions; study hard; prioritize what matters; own up when you don't know; and don't let anyone beat you down – especially that little voice in your own head. If you allow yourself to do it, you'll be amazed by how quickly a new nurse can grow. And I'll be here while you do, lovingly cheering you on.

Real Talk

My hope is that I've uplifted your soul and revived your spirit just in time to bring you crashing back down into the reality that will be your first year (or, sometimes, years) as a newer nurse. The fact of the matter is this: you're going to need a serious support system in order to survive the average days, and an outlet for the even harder ones. My first year as a new graduate nurse in a telemetry unit pales in comparison to the challenges I faced and constant questions buzzing through my brain during my first year in the cardiothoracic intensive care unit. With only thirteen months of experience on the floor, I drugged the director of nursing and forged her signature, therefore granting me an interview to work with arguably the sickest patients in the hospital. Yes, that was a lie, so before anyone threatens to sue me I formally retract my previous statement. But I assure you: that's how it felt! That's how serious this was to me! After witnessing an open-chest code during my clinical as a nursing student, I was transfixed by the idea of working in an environment where adrenaline meets critical thinking and discipline every day. I thought that working in cardiac surgery would be intense: little did I know just how deep the doo-doo I was stepping into would be from my very first shift.

Yes, Doctor

Doctors are very, very good at trying to kill your patients. To the best of my knowledge they aren't intentional in their efforts. Nonetheless, the cornerstone of the nursing profession is protecting the patient lying in bed from becoming the victim of hastiness, sloppiness, or just plain inexperience. Even the newest of bedside nurses can recount the struggles of dealing with a brand new medical resident in the heat of July. While a newly indoctrinated nurse will err on the side of caution, typically asking five million questions and reviewing policies ad nauseum before proceeding to administer medication, perform a procedure, or even order a patient lunch – the first year doctor, sometimes, seems to fall on two ends of a patient care spectrum. Often enough, a new doctor is either shitting her pants with anxiety to the point of total inaction, or she arrogantly dictates orders like the Third Reich.

Please understand one extremely important point: I am by no-means in the business of physician bashing. My very best friend in the world is a physician, and my sister is married to a great one. I have tremendous respect for their passion, practice, and relentless work ethic. Working in the cardiothoracic intensive care unit, I work closely with cardiothoracic surgeons, intensive care physicians, and anesthesiologists who earn every penny they make and then some. They save lives like it's going out of style, and watching them in their practice will leave you awe-struck. I don't ever want you to have chest pain radiating down your left arm…but if you do, my A-team is always ready! However, my public service announcement to anyone who elects to work at a university teaching hospital or big, fat, famous trauma center is this: please encourage your patients to avoid, say, getting hit by a car in July. Got a baby coming that's due on Independence Day? Pray to be induced a week early. Because on July 1st, all across the land, Short-Coats become Long-Coats. Medical students rock a super-obvious short laboratory coat through their training. If you experience this fashion plate, coupled with a shit-eating grin and a terror-filled gaze, there's a pretty good chance that the person holding pressure on your patient's bleeding incision: 1) has never actually done it before; and 2) lied and said she has. I try to be extremely accommodating to medical students in my practice. If they are inquisitive and eager to learn, I do my best to allow them into my patient's room to conduct a head-to-toe examination and, for instance, assist in tasks that require minimally invasive technique. However, foolish be the nurse that lets a student actually *do* something to a patient without circling the room like a hawk! Again, this in no way serves to discredit the medical students and the insane amount of clinical, didactic, and research they undertake: they work their tails off and deserve the best learning experience possible. Just remember that it's your professional license – not theirs – that remains on the line should a task or procedure not according to plan.

Our Short-Coat colleagues generally make a concerted effort to leave a good impression on the nursing staff, and while they want to learn all they can, there are limitations to their practice for practice. Once they graduate from medical school in the spring and start formally training as physicians come summertime, the effort to protect patient safety becomes a more complicated one. The funny part about medical school is it teaches you an awful lot about theory and academia, but usually leaves something to be desired when it comes to actual patient care. A brand spanking new doctor, who must attend medical school, conduct research, volunteer, publish, sell his or her first born child, etcetera – enters a hospital in behind the eight-ball clinically due to the nature of the beast that is medical school. It's residency that takes all of that research and book-learnin'; smashes it into the new resident; forces it to see one, do one, teach one, buy the t-shirt; and do it all over again after thirty-six hours without any sleep. Medical and surgical residency bites the big one, and I am grateful to every medical and surgical resident who has the courage and desire to sacrifice physical and emotional wellbeing for the sake of patient care. However...

Fast forward to Dr. Long-Coat walking through the doors of the hospital. Having earned a medical degree and twelve extra inches of fabric, he or she may feel compelled to prove her worthiness in the hospital setting. From the emergency department to the operating room; from the outpatient facility to the ICU; new residents are worked to the bone physically, mentally, and emotionally. That's where us nurses come in: we often show them what to do, and sometimes, how to do it. We are the best-kept secret for physicians in training. Whether they are a fresh and green first-year intern learning how to order stool softener in the computer system or a third-year surgery resident that needs to crack open a sternum for the first time, we are the high beams that light the dark and winding road toward inevitable screw-upery. Again, I'm not insinuating that physicians are clueless – they absolutely are not. They are brilliant and brave, but they simply lack experience.

So when a seasoned nurse says something like, "Would you like me to start this medication for the patient's heart rate, doctor," it would be foolish to ignore the nuances. Your job – as a newer nurse in any department, every single time – is to follow those cues and learn now to drop hints that can become more than mere suggestions in the future. So much of what you do is in the delivery: you don't enjoy feeling condescended, and I promise you that an overworked and underpaid medical resident would agree. With time you'll learn how to finesse your suggestions and requests in a fashion that protects and promotes the health and safety of your patient, without sounding like a total jerk. Act in a respectful fashion, and you'll be respected in return…most of the time. Sometimes, though, you just sort of have to stiff-arm your way into the order, test, or treatment plan that is most beneficial for your patient. Even if that means being a redundant pain in the ass. Even if that means copping some 'tude. Even if that means – and only under extreme circumstances – threatening to call the attending!

One of the most intense moments I witnessed as a baby nurse in the intensive care unit was during my orientation. When I left my job on the floor for the cardiothoracic ICU, it was safe to say that either I would tread water and stay afloat in order become one of "them," or I would drown and die amid a sea of stressors. (Figuratively "die," of course, in the fashion of, "OMG! Can you believe he said that?! I just died!" *Literal* death as a side effect of a new nursing job, I would imagine, occurs far less frequently.) Of course, as if being the youngest and most inexperienced nurse on the unit wasn't bad enough, I had to thicken my skin; gain my street cred; and study my newbie nurse butt off. I was overwhelmed by the fear that, with me, my new colleagues wouldn't only eat their young: given the entrée, they would lick the plate clean.

On the second to last day of my six-week intensive care nurse whirlwind, where I once again regressed from my position of a pretty good floor nurse to a totally clueless and presumably incompetent ICU one – I realized that there *was* one person who was even more screwed than I was: the surgical resident. He was stocky and sweet; helpful and respectful, but seemed more beta than alpha given the high-stress cardiac surgery environment. This became exceedingly clear when one of the patients developed a really, really low blood pressure – the kind that you would consider incompatible with human life. This patient already had open-heart surgery and was waiting for a bed to go to a step-down unit. I quickly learned that there is no such thing as a stable patient in the ICU. The patient's nurse was preparing the gentleman to transfer upstairs when she noted a massive drop in his blood pressure. If 120/80 is considered textbook normal – cut it in half. That's how low the dude went...and lower...and lower. At first the resident did all the right things: he ordered laboratory work to be drawn to check for any suspicious values; put in for a STAT x-ray of the chest; he even called the patient's surgeon at home on a weekend to notify him of the situation.

When the lab results returned and the x-ray was shot, one of the nurses asked to review the data. This nurse happened to be one of the most bad-ass, hard-ball, patient-saving, adrenaline-loving women I've ever known: a nursing force to be reckoned with. She can be pretty terrifying to new nurses at first, but her intimidation comes from a place of respect for her patients and a passion for her craft. Plus, she just seemed to know everything about everything. It almost became frustrating to work with her because you simply felt inferior while she capably and confidently described patient situations with textbook precision and clinical accuracy. Meanwhile, I was stuck fumbling inside of my mental arsenal for the proper words to formulate a sentence that didn't make me sound like I was suffering from a frontal lobe stroke. A nurse dynamo, this one was – and it turns out, she also happened to be my preceptor. When my veteran dynamo nurse mom (I've had lot's of nurse moms – nurse dads, too!) leaned over the resident's shoulder and peered at the x-ray film, her reaction spoke for itself: "Holy shit, we've gotta' open his chest!" This is not some medical lingo or figure of speech common to nursing practice: *it's a very literal statement*. The patient's x-ray and blood count implied that he was bleeding into his chest cavity, and the only way to save his life was to go back in through his incision, past his ribcage, and into his heart to find – and stop – the source of the bleeding. In situations like this one, time is of the essence. I also learned another valuable pearl of wisdom that morning – bleeding patient responds quite nicely to: 1) receiving blood; and 2) stopping the bleeding (write that tip on a Post-it note, too)! This may seem so simplistic that it borders on stupidity, but it's the truth, and what is *true* is not always what is *easy* for newer nurses.

The heart is like plumbing. It needs blood to pump forward and send oxygen and nutrients to all of the organs and tissues in your body. If the plumbing backs up and blood enters the lungs, a patient has an emergency situation in the form of pulmonary edema. Same goes for a leaky faucet that doesn't stop dripping – a leaky heart valve often results

34

in the need for replacement surgery. Sometimes the plumbing is total crap, and you need the entire fixture replaced – herein lies your heart transplant, the ICU version of a bathroom renovation. In this particular instance, there was no water in the pipes because the pipe had burst and was causing a flood – the patient was bleeding from one of the arteries that was surgically used in bypass, and instead of coursing his blood throughout the body, it was rapidly being pumped into his chest wall.

Holy shit was right! If I thought my very first encounter with a stable patient experiencing 3/10 chest pain a year prior was bad, you could imagine what the prospect of assisting in an open-chest procedure at the bedside was doing to me. As much as I wanted to run to the bathroom to expel my Starbucks, I held strong and stayed in the room. While the tiny-yet-mighty primary nurse hung bags of packed red blood cells, platelets, and fresh frozen plasma quickly and efficiently to replete the patient's dwindling reserve, it became apparent that no quantity of medication was going to save this patient without surgical intervention. Our ICU rooms are all equipped for conversion into full-on operating suites in the event of an emergency. And this – this was the definition of critical.

Although the cardiothoracic surgeon was informed and proceeded to the hospital posthaste, every second of his absence was another moment that a life hung in the balance. (No pressure, though!) To make matters worse, the stout and sweet surgical resident was about to up-chuck all over the room at the sheer thought of managing the escalating situation alone. He didn't look like a deer in headlights – he was way past that point – this poor doc was approaching road kill. When a surgical resident is so flustered that he's frozen in fear, his number one resource isn't a scalpel:

it's a seasoned nurse. My preceptor brought the open chest cart to the doorway – it's literally a filing-cabinet style cart-on-wheels that contains every item one would need for a run-of-the-mill chest cracking. From staples and sutures to a sternal saw reminiscent of a horror film, the open chest cart is the Holy Grail of the cardiothoracic ICU. As an intensive care nurse in training, I placed myself squarely behind the primary nurse managing the patient and watched in awe as my preceptor laid out every required material for the resident. At first hesitant but with skill and focus, the resident proceeded to follow the direct orders from my nurse-mom, looking to her for guidance and reinforcement with every step. With some tough love and a sense of urgency, she adopted a surgical resident as a child, too. From cleaning the patient to creating a sterile environment on which to operate, I was stunned by the vast knowledge, and for what it's worth, the level of importance that every nurse played in this critical situation. Doing the best I could to involve myself in the action without killing anyone or humiliating myself, I stuck to basics: I could verify blood products before they were transfused into the patient, and I could do it damn well. While I labeled and hung bag after bag, the cardiothoracic surgeon rushed into the room and took over the situation. The look on the resident's face was a combination of relief and panic that seemed to shout, "Thank God he's here! Where is the nearest bathroom?!" With some persistence and an occasional f-bomb, the attending surgeon was immediately able to localize the source of the patient's bleed and correct the problem with suture and cautery. And wouldn't ya know it? All bleeding really does stop eventually! The patient recovered without incident and was sent upstairs the next day, anyone not involved none the wiser to his brush with death twenty-four hours prior. Me, though? I'm not sure that I'll ever recover from that day...from that moment. It was the first time in my life, as a born-again baby nurse, that it became crystal-clear that there is no such thing as "just a nurse." Nurses are the silent benefactors that enrich the lives of patients and physicians alike. Nurses keep you happy. Nurses keep you comfortable. Most importantly – while they rarely take the credit – nurses keep you alive.

Mad Skills

The head-to-toe assessment is one of those rites of nursing passage that separates the unsure nursing student from the still unsure yet legally licensed novice nurse. Truth be told, not much changes. You're going to start your first shift and wonder how the hell it's possible to assess one (or four or five or ten) patients thoroughly; keep breath sounds and intravenous lines and skin conditions straight between patients; adequately document all of this every few hours; and actually make it out of work before your next shift starts! If you only have a few minutes to devote to each patient at the start of your shift, be sure to create a general assessment that encompasses multiple pieces at once, and then hone in on a focused assessment based on why the patient has presented to the hospital. For example, if your patient was admitted for a congestive heart failure exacerbation, focus on heart and lung sounds; skin color, temperature and presence of edema; even urine output reflective of renal function or diuresis. In a stroke patient, a focused neurological assessment is key. If you're in the ICU, you're going to have to focus your assessment on every inch of the person in that bed – it's best to tackle one patient in a stepwise approach and maintain consistency in your assessments to follow every time. For example, I assess all of my patients using the following pattern: *Neuro, pupils, motor, pain, respiratory, cardiac, gastrointestinal, genitourinary, pulses, skin, access, endocrine, and infectious disease.*

Every patient. Every time. Whether I'm assessing my patient or conducting morning rounds or handing off at the end of my shift, I am religiously reciting that pattern in my head. When I was a new graduate nurse on the floor and had five patients to assess, I would use a quick and dirty version of the same method with my daily patient load. While you cant take up the entire morning assessing one patient, it is critical that you actually look, listen, and feel. You may receive handoff at the start of your shift from Super Nurse who always has her shift life together. You might even feel compelled to trust her assessment instead of your own. Nip that habit in the bud the moment it enters your brainwaves. I don't care if the Chief Nursing Officer of the hospital tells you that your patient has a twenty gauge peripheral IV with beautiful blood return that doesn't expire until tomorrow. You go into that room: look, touch, and flush the hell out of that line; and you conduct your own assessment – every patient, every time.

Just as important as actually assessing your patient – (think skin, people! Pressure ulcers hide between the cheeks, so crack that behind like a walnut and get in there!) – is evaluating the patient care environment. Imagine entering you patient's room at the start of your shift and seeing linens, dirty food trays, and dressing materials strewn about. Your job in that moment is not to blame the previous nurse (although I promise you every one of us has been chewed out for housekeeping matters before). Instead, you are to quickly and efficiently create a safe practice environment for yourself and for your patient. Those chairs the family left at the bedside? Blocking your Ambu-Bag. The patient tray table sitting in the middle of the room? Occluding a fire exit. And if you patient was to unexpectedly code – flat out, point blank, cardiac arrest – where could you possibly fit a code cart and the forty other people that come along with it?

It wasn't until I became an ICU nurse that I was trained to be so keenly aware of my patient's environment of care, and how those physical obstacles might become literal barriers to saving a life. Assessing your patient's safety is tantamount, and any nurse will quickly learn how important that can be the first time his or her patient experiences a forbidden fall on the way to the bathroom. Always conduct the assessment that your nursing instructor would have wanted for SIM Man. Phone a friend and get another set of eyeballs if you see, hear, or smell something that doesn't quite seem right to you. And for the love of God, straighten up after yourself – you don't work in a barn, you know! Unless, of course, you happen to know a farmer with a medical emergency…

If You Didn't Document it...

To be fair, as a novice nurse, you probably didn't have enough time to do it! But as the old nursing adage goes, "If you didn't document it, you didn't do it!" Never will that sentence mean more to you than in a court of law; sitting on the stand; being deposed for something that came up regarding a patient you cared for many years prior. You probably won't have a goddamn clue what the attorney is even talking about, and while you might be inclined to defend yourself – in that very moment, whatever is charted in your patient's record is the only evidence admissible in a court of law.

As a corporate slave before becoming a nurse, the prospect of legality in nursing has always been something that I've been keenly aware of – no matter how large or small, what you write in your patient's record can (and will) be used against you in a court of law. With that said, it is in your best interest to only document what you see; what you do; who you call; and situations that arise. Be cautious of leaving out every detail, as omitting a progress note or narrative may position you with no proof of a task done, med given, or dressing changed, for example. On the flipside, over-documenting can be detrimental to your patient record as well. Many institutions have veered away from paper documentation. This conversion toward computer charting seems to allow for a veil of anonymity and disconnect between what you can type in a small box and what actually occurs. Every time you save your password in that digital flow sheet, you are creating a legally binding electronic signature that holds equal weight to a pen and paper John Hancock. Wham. Bam. Thank you, ma'am.

Understand that the nursing scope is very different from one of a physician, and documentation of actual medical diagnoses is not the same thing as creating a nursing care plan with nursing diagnoses. Whether your day was dull and ordinary or filled with chaos and catastrophe, make sure that your documentation is thorough, consistent, and your own work before you click save. If you didn't document it, you can't take credit; if you over share information, you may dig yourself into a hole where you'll remain. Follow the only nurse rule that can be applied to wearing a mini-skirt: it should be short enough to get to the point, and long enough to cover the important stuff, all while keeping you out of trouble.

One final note: I was encouraged immediately upon becoming a licensed registered nursing professional to purchase my own malpractice insurance. While it's true that your institution will likely provide some form of coverage to you as an employee, I cannot emphasize enough the importance of properly protecting yourself and your practice. Even if you're the most thorough and competent clinician on the planet, the universe doesn't always work in ways that are logical, sensible, or theoretical: shit happens. Given the peace of mind it affords, your own insurance plan is one hundred dollars very well spent.

Up Above the Cloud

One of the most crucial resources you'll come to rely on, as a nurse at every level in today's day and age, is the Internet. You can walk into any kindergarten classroom these days and see children handling tablets and smartphones with greater ease and dexterity than your parents. This is a digital age, my friends, and one must be aware of the great and powerful Cloud. If you survived nursing school anytime in the last decade, you're already familiar with the tools and resources available through technology – especially when it comes to finding alternatives to learning that extend beyond just picking up a book and reading. In fact, some of the tools that not only aided in my initial foray into nursing, but also were crucial in helping me acclimate to an ICU environment, can be found at the touch of a button.

First and foremost, just passing my nursing boards required the help of a question bank application that I downloaded onto my smartphone. For fifteen or so bucks, I had access to over one thousand questions pertaining to every category that would be covered on the NCLEX. The best part about this method was the convenience: I could sit in the break room at work before my patient care technician shift and take a short quiz, or I could walk on the treadmill while learning about dreaded obstetric emergencies or the difference between a PTT and an INR. Frankly, I had no excuse to be unprepared: I was no longer liable for lugging giant textbooks around with me for rote memorization and review. I'll admit that everyone has their own preferred method of study – mine happens to be reading and recall – but I guarantee that whether you are cramming for one exam or learning about your specialized practice, there are digital resources that will serve in your favor.

When I entered the cardiothoracic intensive care unit, the quantity of information I would be expected to digest and regurgitate seemed astounding. Coming from a non-ICU background, I could feel my inner model student start to panic – how the hell was I expected to learn the basic tenets of critical care, and recover fresh post-surgical patients, *and* anticipate clinical emergencies, all without killing a patient on my very first day alone? All I can say is thank the Nursing Gods for my iPhone! Numerous nursing applications – some even specific to cardiothoracic surgery – gave me everything a newbie nurse could need, ranging from body systems to hemodynamics to pharmacology to medical and surgical emergencies. These resources were well worth the cost, as I can think back to countless evenings when I reflected on morning rounds and thought to myself, "What the hell are they talking about?" With a few clicks and a couple dollars, I was able to review and reinforce content in order to pace my conceptual understanding to my clinical abilities.

Additionally, there were countless mega-awesome websites that I stumbled upon in my incessant search for "ICU for Dummies" materials. Through free nursing driven websites, I could conveniently peruse topics like EKG interpretation, chest tube drains, and ventilators for beginners. Trust me, whether you're new nurse in critical care or never plan to set foot in an intensive care unit for your entire career, the insights and nursing wisdom that are available to the public for free is outrageous! I've spent hours on YouTube watching cardiac surgery; on Google Scholar reading abstracts and articles; and on nurse-driven websites learning how to incorporate my new-found knowledge into practice.

Finally, though crazy it may be, I swear by the power of social media in serving as a resource to learn and grow in your practice. I'm serious! It's not all #selfies and self-promotion. With the right social network – be it Facebook, Instagram, Twitter, or Pinterest, among others – you can learn information, read articles and research, and share questions and concerns with fellow nursing compatriots. In fact, some of the most interesting and useful mnemonics about anatomy, pathophysiology, and pharmacology were sourced from social media networks. As an added bonus, you can score a good laugh by checking out some of the ridiculous jokes, photos, and videos that your fellow nurses and nursing students concoct in a desperate effort to procrastinate from whatever task is currently at hand. My point is this: the Internet is full of quacks, hackers, trolls, and super-scary content, and you should never let your practice be cat-fished! However, when appropriately sourced, referenced, and utilized, it can be the quickest and most effective path from point A to point B. When point A is a state of complete and utter cluelessness, one wants to progress to point B pretty freaking quickly! Embrace how technology has impacted your education; recognize that will only continue to grow as a necessity in your nursing practice; and remember to use the power of the Cloud for good and not evil.

Don't #SELFIE Yourself Short

I have a confession to make: I'm something of a selfie queen. Some might say that my social media game is strong, and that I have followers who range from my great aunt to total strangers. We live in a digital age where social media connects us, markets us, and in many ways defines us. But before you post that Facebook status or tweet that photograph, think before you link. All it takes is one bonehead public post or picture to jeopardize your nursing career and even your professional license. If you know that we live in a world where someone could Google you while they are sitting on the can, why would you ever publicize anything that could come back to haunt you in the future?

My point blank, straight up, first and foremost rule of social media is this: if I couldn't delete this, would it impact me in any way? It's so easy to show the world what we are up to at the precise second that we're doing it – that doesn't mean your boss should be privy to that information. As a matter of fact, there are institutions across the country that adhere employees to strict "no social media" policies. As crazy as that might sound – especially to someone like myself, who frequents social media daily as a valuable tool– logic would dictate that someone did something really, really stupid for such a policy to be enacted.

Simple common sense is a wonderful tool in deciding what is appropriate to be posted to the public, and what should remain locked away and hidden in a box under your bed. You are 100% entitled to your opinions, as long as said opinions don't in any way violate HIPPA or read as libel toward your place of employment. You are generally allowed to snap a selfie, as long as that photo doesn't contain patient information or take place in the heat of a unit-based emergency. You can absolutely brag about that autograph you scored from Peyton Manning, as long as the quarterback wasn't your patient…and said "autograph" isn't the signature on his discharge instructions. And you can definitely check into the cool new bar in town on Facebook, as long as you didn't call out of work sick to attend the opening. You see, my friend – it's so easy! And yet for many of us, it's still harder than the passing pharmacology. When that patient comes in with a crazy rash or a gnarly mangled appendage or some weird-as-hell mystery diagnosis, resist the urge to pull the iPhone out of your pocket – given your position, you very well may be Snap Chatting your way to the unemployment line.

So You Killed Your
First Patient

Fine, hopefully you only *thought* you killed your first patient. Unfortunately, whether it's feeding a patient who is scheduled for a procedure or giving the incorrect dose of stool softener, there's going to come a moment when you screw up. The most important rule of patient safety as a novice nurse entering the hospital world translates across every type of unit: *always* be sure of how to do something before you do it. If you've never administered a particular antibiotic before, be certain to call the pharmacy and ask about how it should be infused. If you've never placed a nasogastric tube in a vomiting patient, absolutely confirm your hospital policy regarding tube placement verification and management. The list of what you must do and how you should do it can go on ad nauseam, but you absolutely positively should never-ever-freaking-ever do something that you don't feel comfortable doing. Establishing responsible habits early in your career, and checking yourself as you progress, will help you avoid mishaps and errors during those particularly crazy, full-moon, emergency room exploding, a billion ICU holds kind of shifts.

I'll never forget being a brand-new ICU nurse and receiving my first phone call at home from work. It was nearly ten o'clock in the evening. I had already entered the first phase of the REM cycle, when the buzzing on my bedside table startled me to a state of sheer panic. I was convinced – absolutely and utterly convinced – that I had killed my sick patient and was being notified that I'd been fired. Every nurse's first thought isn't, "Are you interested in working overtime tomorrow?" It's more along the lines of, "Dear God, I've done it…this is it, it's time to clean out my locker." It turns out my mistake was an error in charting a dosage, not in the actual dose of medication that the patient was receiving. Nonetheless, from that very moment I swore that every last iota of my documentation would be as buttoned-up as possible. This wasn't a near miss. It certainly wasn't a sentinel event. However, it stuck with me because of the ten million possibilities that swirled around my weary mind when that telephone rang. Nurses in general are responsible for so many varied tasks, and our licenses are contingent upon the idea that we do no harm. Just the idea of unintentionally causing harm to a patient can be enough to scare any nurse straight. Pause, think, and reflect before you provide any sort of care, even when and *especially if* you are extremely busy: the safety and well being of your patient – and your professional license – depend on it.

Unfortunately, to err is human: there may come a time when something very bad does happen to one of your patients, and you are the one held responsible for the cause and effect. Own up to your error, and be honest and forthcoming the moment that you recognize that something you did could bring harm to the person under your care. Perhaps you inserted a latex urinary catheter into someone with an allergy. Maybe you accidentally gave the wrong insulin varietal. Heaven forbid you administered the wrong blood product to a bleeding patient – but in the history of nursing practice it's has happened before, and no doubt, it will happen again. Own up to what you've done, and make it a priority to provide supportive care to remedy the situation as soon as possible. If this all sounds super scary as a baby nurse, understand that it doesn't become any less so as a seasoned one. Experienced nurses mess up too, and they are equally as liable and responsible as you with your brand new license. Nursing is 24/7: I know that you've heard this over and over again during school, and you'll continue to hear it until you're sick and tired of the phrase throughout your career. It's true. It's consistent. And it matters. Don't let shortcuts, a busy assignment, or fear of nurse-to-nurse handoff pigeonhole you into making stupid decisions at the expense of your patient. Treat every patient the way you would want to be treated – especially those who may not be able to speak or advocate for themselves. This will not only save you a mistake headache, it could very well save you a deposition in a courtroom.

Indecent Exposure

You're going to see more penis than a brothel, and more vagina than a George Clooney look-alike gynecologist. You'll poke more backsides than a creepy guy on the subway, and get flashed more than a Girls Gone Wild video. And you'll get paid to do it, too! This, my baby nurse friends, simply comes with the territory. There are absolutely areas of nursing where you can deal with fully clothed patients on the regular, but the hospital is not one of them. Even if you have a totally stable walkie-talkie admission, you're going to have to thoroughly assess their bodies as part of your care. You could have a Calvin Klein model in your hospital bed, and you'll *still* have to properly cleanse the urethral meatus. How terrible would it be if you let your lack of professionalism get in the way of your job, and the heartthrob underwear model gets a CAUTI because you were too flustered to glove up and wipe down? (For baby nurses who are unfamiliar with the term "CAUTI," I suggest you memorize it now: Catheter Acquired Urinary Tract Infection – the bane of all hospital systems!)

If this all sounds ludicrous, I promise you that I have a point: it's your job to provide the same level of care to every patient, in all situations. There might be moments when patients feel uncomfortable allowing you to render care because you're too young or too handsome or have cold hands or refuse to wear gloves. Whatever the case may be, it's important that you educate your patient regarding the necessity of assessment as it pertains to their health, and that you're professionally trained to go boldly where no nurse has gone before. If they still refuse – and to be fair, they have the right too – you should offer up a different nurse or nursing assistant to assist with the task. Some hospitals, for instance, have a two-nurse policy when inserting urinary catheters not only to ensure adherence to sterile technique, but also to allow the patient the presence of another person during the uncomfortable act.

One other important point of note is something that probably became apparent during nursing school: you're going to encounter lots of interesting elements of human anatomy and physiology as a baby nurse, and it only becomes more fascinating as your career progresses. Remember that the person in that bed is a human being who deserves to be treated with respect and dignity. Instead of declaring to another nurse, "I just finished cleaning so-and-so and he pooped all over again," choose your words and expressions in a professional and respectful manner. Even if a patient claims that everyone's "already seen it all anyway," be conscientious about maintaining their decency: limit exposure to areas as needed; cover your patient up as quickly as possible; and always close curtains and doors before rendering care. Further, as a patient advocate, you should always ensure that physicians and medical staff entering your patient room adhere to the same standards. The simple act of drawing the shades or closing a curtain can make the world of difference to a patient enduring a clinical procedure or a delicate conversation. You're going to have plenty of patients who insist on exposing their bits to you intentionally. If you develop your sense of decency before that time comes, you won't be blindsided by a surprise when you run into the room and catch your patient relieve the stressors of being hospitalized with five fingers and artifact on the telemetry monitor!

PART II:

OH SHIT! NOBODY TAUGHT
ME THIS IN SCHOOL!
Mean Girls (And Guys)

I wish I could tell you that new nurses are always coddled, hugged, beloved, and nurtured into becoming incredible men and women that shape the future of nursing as a whole. But I would clearly be drunk or delusional, and I've resigned myself to strictly one glass of red wine per chapter of this book. So I might be buzzed, but I'm absolutely not crazy. There exist numerous personalities in the nursing world that every nurse encounters, and some are far more damaging to the newbie nurse psyche than others. I have made it a point to maintain a sense of pride for my profession and respect for my colleagues since my very first day setting foot on a hospital floor, yet there will always be people that you can simply never please. Even if you're the smartest, most organized, efficient nurse in the entire planet – in general – there's going to be that one nurse who believes being a clueless and sloppy is the preferred evidence-based practice. I'm not telling you to grow a thick skin – but definitely realize that you're going to need a callus or two to survive the nature of the nursing beast.

I've been called ditzy, dumb, and blonde. I've been too pretty, too plastic, and have obviously been chasing surgeons. I've been too happy and too high-energy and too rosy when I should be, perhaps, miserable, drab, and dreary gray. I can go on and on about why the concept of nurses eating their young is poor practice and promotes a hostile work environment, but I promise the topic has been beaten to death and I am no expert on the matter. All I can offer you, short of some anecdotal advice and a big fat theoretical eff-you to anybody who might get in your way, is the encouragement to prove every last one of the bullies wrong through your actions. Truth be told, I've never understood why the profession seems to allow the practice of scaring novice nurses into submission for decades on end. In part it seems like a sorority-esque sub-culture derived from an, "I survived the hazing, now you must too," mentality. Whether the female dominance in the profession adds to the flavor of being made to feel belittled, berated, or backstabbed by colleagues is uncertain to me, although numerous males in nursing experience this struggle just the same. What's important to remember as you transition from a new nurse and grow more experienced is that nurse-bullies don't know what to do once they've been stood up to: first they become confused; then they're sort of pissed-off; and finally they retreat. While they may seem to enjoy making you feel like the bottom of the totem pole, once you assert yourself in a manner that shows you've got the confidence to support your practice and stand up for yourself through it all, they will likely back down and shy away. Whether this is some annoyingly archaic rite of passage or just a sense of insecurity regarding a power shift, novice nurses who succeed in assertively yet respectfully standing up to confrontation are eventually accepted as members of the team. If this sounds utterly bat-shit crazy, it's because it is just that: completely and totally insane. I don't want to leave you with the idea that you should accept this practice because it's the way it's always been – in fact; one of my biggest motivators in writing a book for new nurses is to help them stand up for their practices and principles. However, the evolution of this archaic remnant of nursing past seems to be slower than suits the profession. If we want to be treated like an ethical and compassionate group of healthcare providers, it would stand to reason that we treat one another with ethics and compassion. Nonetheless, there are levels of this dynamic in every profession – the ones who work as nurses simply happen to feel justified in their belittling nature, and herein lies the problem that only effective practice, respectful assertiveness, and an occasional "screw you" attitude seem to temporarily fix. Is this a good solution to a disturbingly deep-seated problem? No: it's a terrible way to manage what threatens the personal and professional satisfaction of those entering the nursing domain. Should we encourage one another to only look down on someone when lending a hand to lift them up? Absolutely. Is this nursing utopia even possible given the stressors and struggles that nurses face in their work every single day? Call me an eternally glass half-full kinda gal, but I believe it reasonable to think that educated members of society who are praised for being the cornerstone of integrity by and large across the world possess a capacity to stop being so damn mean. Remember this when you're an older and wiser nurse someday, and you see a new baby nurse that is struggling to find his or her bearings. Multiple acts of kindness and encouragement will *probably* be remembered – but make no mistake about it, one horrible hazing moment will *never* be forgotten.

If the going gets tougher than you had expected and you are truly feeling threatened at the workplace, your job is to open your mouth and speak up. If the nurse-bullying tactics remain even after having a colleague-to-colleague discussion, it's time to advance the issue to your nurse manager or beyond. I can't reiterate this enough: just because something is happening the way it always has, doesn't mean it's the way it needs to always be. Stand up for yourself; be clear in your intentions; protect yourself and your practice; and don't let your novice status make you feel inferior. You're already a vital resource for patients, physicians, and nurse colleagues: someday you'll genuinely recognize it. No matter the circumstances, allow yourself to be Cady Heron in a world littered with Regina Georges. Mean Girls (and Guys) have their place in the movies – not in the halls of a hospital. And you, Glenn Coco? You go, Glenn Coco!

Be Nice to Everyone

There is no question that a hospital feels like one of the final vestiges of society where hierarchy and rank still reign supreme. Whether it's the steps required of a medical student before becoming an attending or the role of a nursing assistant that must climb through the ranks toward nursing autonomy, there are multiple levels within layers in an acute care setting. And much like a literal onion, this hospital onion may leave you in tears. You're going to feel like you're at the very bottom of the theoretical totem pole as a new nurse, and this might incite you to take it out on those ancillary folks in roles outside of your own. My suggestion is you do everything in your power to maintain grace, class, and a sense of respect for every person you come into contact with professionally. You might work your way from the role of a novice in the field to an expert status: this doesn't allow you to look down upon or act with disrespect toward any of the other participants of the patient care experience who are down in the trenches with you.

I want you to repeat after me: *I am not above the role of nursing assistant. I am not above the role of housekeeper or host. I am not above the role of food service provider. I am not above the role of engineering. I am not above the pharmacists, respiratory therapists, physical therapists, occupational therapists, or speech language pathologists. They (and so very many more) are all committed to the progress and improvement of my patient care.*

Like wise, I want you to chant this in the mirror: *I am not beneath an attending physician…figuratively speaking.   I am not beneath a surgeon. I am not beneath an executive or a nurse manager or the vice president of anything.   I am not beneath my advanced practice professionals and physician's assistants. I am not beneath an intern, a resident, or a fellow. I aim to provide the highest level of competent and compassionate care, and I am a part of the team that is required to deliver the greatest possible service to those charged with my nursing practice.*

You will likely progress through your time as a baby nurse believing that you've been disrespected, belittled, or made to feel inferior in some capacity. A natural inclination when this happens may be to pass that horrible feeling along to others. Resist the urge. If you treat your ancillary help like trash, odds are, they will remember and reflect on this. Conversely, if you take on any role and assist whenever possible, there is a pretty good chance that anybody outside of the nursing realm will be happy to interact with you on a daily basis. My first job in a hospital during nursing school was as a patient care technician: I never worked so hard as when I did in this role. While nurses are responsible for providing care to a handful (sometimes more than a handful, I know) of patients, a nursing assistant might have to take on an entire department by his or herself. Not only does this role require flexibility, time management, and compassion toward patients in some of their darkest moments, you are also being pulled in every direction by nursing staff looking for a boost, turn, lift, or refresher. The same could be said for every ancillary partner that you work with – the fact of the matter is, while your job is super freaking hard, they make you look good!

By the same token, your advanced practice nurses and physician's assistants are often going to be a direct link between you and the physician who is assigned to your patient. They can be some of the greatest resources and most skillful clinicians you ever come across – I still have moments when I'm baffled by some of the amazing things I get to see when an APN or PA-C gets down and dirty inside of an open chest during a messy code. While they are technically "above" you in terms of position, these folks depend on the insight and critical thinking of the nurse caring for their patients. They will rely on you as the eyes and ears of your patient condition, and so very much of what you need in the way of orders, procedures, emotional support, and beyond can be acquired through a thoughtful conversation with your advanced practice team. The dynamic here goes the same way with any other cohorts of employees that you interact with outside of the nursing bubble: if you scratch their backs through well thought-out interactions, they will come to utilize you as a point of reference for their patient care. I really hope this all feels like a series of common sense, "no shit, Sherlock" moments – but the fact that I feel driven to put the Golden Rule into effect means that it might not be as clear-cut and easy-peasy as it seems on the surface. When you're stressed out; pissed off; hungry; angry; hangry; or running around like a lunatic, being a levelheaded team player might be at the bottom of your to-do list. If that's the case, simply take the list out of one of your many cargo pockets; tear it to shreds; and reorganize your nursing priorities.

The OG's

The greatest reference guide for a new nurse may have nothing to do with a reference guide, iPhone app, or online nursing forum. Rather, it comes from the brain of a highly experienced, done it all, seen it all, experienced nurse. There's a very strange dynamic when you work in a setting that is peppered with nurses at every stage of their career. Some are much like you – new to the game, unsure and uncertain of every step along the way. Others have progressed; found their groove and make everything look natural. And that final cohort – the sage; the wise; the nurses who remain cool and calm despite the fire lit under their proverbial asses – they are a special gift in this profession. Allow them to guide you through your uncertainty, for they have been there, done that, and bought the "oh shit" T-shirt.

Veteran nurses came into this profession long before computer charting and advanced medical technology. They are a rare breed of professionals who were trained to assess patients thoroughly and strictly by their own eyes, ears, and healing hands. Without assistive devices and bedside technologies and invasive monitors to do the work for them, this crop of nurses can predict that your patient is going into heart failure, pulmonary edema, or becoming septic long before the test results come back. And yet somehow, for whatever reason, the basis of their inherent practice seems to be diminished and downplayed in favor of modern evidence-based techniques and standards. I don't for a second wish to demean progress – healthcare has evolved in such a way that technology and research is finally shaping the way that nurses practice. I do, however, believe that it's ridiculous and insulting to disregard decades of experience and professional clinical judgment for the sake of an isolated lab result or a number on a monitor. We are so quick to jump to conclusions based on what technology dictates that we often miss the point of the overall clinical picture. Veteran nurses don't focus in on just one color of a patient canvas. While new nurses clinically color by numbers, seasoned nurses have the experience and insight to view the entire pixelated situation and extract meaning from the nuances.

Next time you are at the hospital and working with nurses who have perhaps been practicing for more years than you've been on this planet, do yourself a favor and take the time to observe them. Hang onto every word that passes their lips: from how they start the shift in a patient room to how they conduct hand off to another nurse at the end of the day. You might be pleasantly surprised to find that an experienced nurse might be the most valuable resource to a doctor on your floor. You may be delighted to know that he or she does more than simply judge current practice or performance – in fact, she has had to adapt to the changes in technique and shifts in paradigm for decades. And you might be shocked to know that what you've mistaken for burnout or a jaded sense is actually a realistic perspective and a snarky sense of humor. These are two components of the complex nursing puzzle that serve as protective mechanisms to allow the wiser members of the nursing community to AEPIE the hell out of patients for shift after shift.

As a new to practice nurse, you should learn to recognize the veteran nurses who have paved the way for you in your clinical practice; the ones who fought for their patients and family members; the ones who have served as a shoulder to cry on for the stressed out staff, and as a brain to pick for inquisitive practitioners. Even if it feels like hierarchical poppycock, respecting the OG's of nursing is a sure-fire way to help you bridge the gap between newbie nurse insecurities and evolving nurse certainty.

"Murses:" Could We Not!

For whatever reason, I've taken some heat in the past for not including male nurses into my writing. The use of "she" as a universal pronoun apparently screws with peoples heads, and therefore I've received comments and complaints in my previous works about leaving dudes out of the nursing equation. Let me make a few things perfectly clear: first, I opt to use the universal "she" in my work because, frankly, it just sounds better than dropping a "he/she" bomb all over my sentence structure. It's purely grammar meets aesthetic. Secondly, when I write thoughts, feelings, and emotions from my own perspective – and I do, indeed, possess the requisite lady-bits to place me in the "she" category – this is not to discredit the fact that men and women alike can relate to what I have gone through as a new nurse and beyond. And finally – this is something I know to be true not only in my blogs and articles but across a whole spectrum of social, political, and pop cultural issues: *people need to lighten the f*ck up.* I'm not sure when our society lost focus on issues that truly require deep thought and introspection and opted to focus on turning minutiae into mayhem, but apparently it occurs often enough that I feel obligated to preface my position toward men in nursing with evidence that I'm neither an anti-feminist nor am I a man-basher. I love men and women equally: it's the assholes of the world that I struggle to embrace.

So, now that I've successfully disclosed any conflicts of gender interest, I can dive into how men in this profession shake up the nursing experience. Whether you are a male nurse or happen to work with one, dudes in nursing (who I refuse to call "murses" – a nurse is a nurse is a nurse, whether you have P or a V anything in between. And doesn't "murse" mean "man purse" anyway?! At least that's what Urban Dictionary taught me...) add balance to what has potential to be a lopsided work environment. Comprising less than ten percent of the profession in the United States as a whole, this staggering statistic makes it surprising that you would encounter men in nursing during your career at all! And yet in my current role in the CTICU, I work with so many male colleagues that you could create an entire "Men of Cardiac Surgery" calendar. I don't hope to treat my nursing bros as pieces of man-meat, however, so I'll stick to utilizing them for their intended purpose: lifting help and poop jokes. (I kid. It's a joke. Lighten the f*ck up.)

As a brand-new nurse, acclimating to a stressful and dynamic work environment is difficult to begin with. Being a new *male* nurse – well, that comes with its own set of challenges. The stereotypes that pervade the nursing profession are ones that, quite frankly, seem to embody more "feminine" qualities: nurturing; caring; compassion; selflessness. Likewise, emotional labiality, cattiness, subservience, and passive-aggressiveness all come to mind as the flip side of these attributes. So where do males come into play? How can a gender that is widely expected to present as "strong and silent" or "tough and gruff" or "adrenaline-loving daredevils" expect to parlay into a profession that seems to be teeming with feminine influences – good, bad, and ugly? And are these roles as strictly defined, as they once appeared to be?

Well my own experience has flipped conventional stereotypes on its head, then spun it around backwards just for good measure. As a newbie male nurse, you don't need to enter your role confined by antiquated archetypes of the profession. Interestingly, it turns out that Florence Nightingale – the mother of nursing herself – preferred to keep the company of powerful and intelligent men! Her biography teaches us that she eventually went on to die alone as a decrepit spinster, but that says nothing of her desire to surround herself with thinkers that expanded the traditional concept of "nursing" outside of its prim and proper, white starched box. Male nurses – whether new to the role or seasoned veterans in practice – possess the capacity to deliver compassionate, patient-centered care on par with females in the profession...many times, even more so. If we're pulling statistics, the numbers indicate that male nurses gravitate towards critical care and the emergency department in greater quantities than female nurses do, and perhaps that allows them to practice in a capacity that showcases their supposed "inherent" strengths without being plagued by endless insufferable "Gaylord Focker" references.

Male baby nurses, you are going to have certain scenarios play out that seem to be universal struggles for men in nursing. You're going to walk into a patient room – maybe even on your very first day in a hospital – and be mistaken for a doctor. The patient or family member guilty of this mix-up will proceed to assault you with a series of awkward questions. They might apologize for the confusion, and offer a backhanded compliment about how nurses are *so important* to patient care. Perhaps they will ask you why you became a became a nurse instead of attending medical school, and despite your perfectly rational and appropriate response, you'll spend the remainder of your shift feeling inadequate, offended, or just plain crappy. It's not that you're embarrassed to be a nurse – far from it! You worked your tail off during nursing school; studied hard to pass your boards; overcame the interview process; and earned your spot with the best of them. The struggle that seems to be more apparent in new male nurses than their female colleagues is the sense that they must justify every element of their nursing practice. If you study nursing in college, the roasting, joking, and judgment seems to be stifled by bragging rights on a ten-to-one chick-to-bro ratio. If you work on a medical unit, there is pressure to move into a more dynamic and complex department. If you work in the trenches as a staff nurse, there is the expectation that you'll return to school and become an advanced practice something-or-other. If you are content in your role and comfortable with your career, there is an assumption that you're bound by the constraints of your personal life – or worse yet (GASP) – that your significant other is the breadwinner/ head of household/ wears the pants in the relationship. These circumstances aren't hard and fast rules across the board – this profession contains three million plus members in the United States alone, so there is no way I can speak for everyone in every setting. But I wouldn't be surprised if you as a male novice nurse battle a stressful inner dialogue that asks not only that you defend your own practice and clinical expertise, but your identity as well.

So much of the pressure that falls upon males in nursing is self-inflicted, and gaining confidence in your clinical abilities and social interactions will help you work through the insecurities and evolve into a calm and collected member of the nursing team. Of course, don't be surprised if you're monopolized for lifting, turning, and boosting help along the way! As a matter of fact, there can be a tendency for other nurses to take advantage of your apparent brut strength: even if you're 110 pounds soaking wet, the fact that you're male will turn you into a turn and reposition target! Being a team-player and helping your colleagues isn't the same as being taken advantage of – don't be afraid to ask for help when you need it; say no when you must; and protect your own practice before you lend yourself to others.

It goes without saying that many of my best friends and most respected colleagues in the workplace are males. Working with male colleagues has afforded me more than a bevy of intelligent work husbands who are there when I need them most (namely, while tackling a monumental fecal incident) – and whether proverbial or literal shit hits the fan, they are always among the first on the scene to stabilize the patient and offer assistance. They have encouraged me to work beyond my baseline level of practice through their clinical insights, professional camaraderie, and general ability to remain levelheaded during the most emotionally trying times. This doesn't imply that they don't take the work home with them, however. They admittedly feel shaken up by the especially challenging shifts, and often become emotional when a meaningful patient experiences a difficult upset or an inspirational victory. The biggest thank you I owe my male nurse brothers from another mother is simple: they are direct; they are efficient; and they prove their prowess through their practice. One can hope to expect a day with low levels of drama, high quantities of laughter, and a constant helping hand. So to the male newbie male nurses out there who, despite perhaps being too embarrassed to admit it, are shitting your pants at the thought of functioning independently, capably, and comfortably: trust me, your time will come. Take pride in how far you've progressed, and be excited about where you're going. The journey to nursing greatness takes time, discipline, and dependence on those who've been there and done that before you were around. Know when to man up, as the saying goes, and when to let others take the lead. In due time, my friend, you'll make that asshole Jack Byrnes and his precious Jinxie cat your bitch.

PART III

OH SHIT! I'M FEELING THE FEELS
You'll Always Remember Your First

I'll always remember my first.

It hurt. A lot. He was in his eighties, and his name was Joseph. It was uncomfortable nearly to the point of unbearable, but I made it through the cold and gray afternoon. I survived the experience, and I was a changed woman because of it. Every nurse remembers his or her first patient death. I've seen dozens and dozens of patients die since that chilly November afternoon, but I will always remember Joe as the one who shaped how I would respond to these moments in the future.

Most people don't go to work and see dead people. Most people have careers that might be challenging and interesting, exciting and on the cutting edge, but generally speaking, nobody dies from an unanswered email. That is the thing about being a critical care nurse that has both helped me find perspective in some situations, and frustrated the hell out of me during others. There will come a time as a nurse – whether you are brand new or have some solid experience under your belt – that you will lose someone. It might be a dramatic code blue made for television drama, or it could be a planned transition with a morphine drip and a grieving family at the bedside. No matter the circumstance, there is nothing that will prepare for that day when it comes. You're going to take it all in – every amp of epi you might have pushed; every fragment of rib you compressed; every drop of fluid you administered – that's going to circulate within you for a while…and this is totally normal. New nurses walk into their roles with the understanding that *well* people don't frequent the hospital: *sick* ones do. But there's something so raw and real about seeing a human being take their last breath – no amount of studying will ever teach you how to feel or think in that very moment. When I lost my first patient, it was something of a planned event. He was elderly; had multiple chronic issues; and decided that he had fought as much as he was willing to fight. Joe drifted off peacefully into the afterlife while his children surrounded him.

When I compare that experience to my first loss in the ICU, the clinical picture couldn't be more of a polar opposite. The bleeding and coding and compressing and screaming have left a permanent imprint in my brain. It's been locked away in my nursing arsenal along with a laundry list of things I felt that were in my control, and others that I only could have dreamed to understand. My first post-surgical bloody ugly code made me feel like a useless member of the surgical team. I blamed myself for the fact that my patient came out with a surgical complication; one that could only have been fixed through sternal re-exploration. Although I held my own and tried to titrate medications and hang blood products as quickly and safely as possible, my baby nurse reserve was very quickly depleted. After coding the patient back into the operating room and hearing a few hours later that he died on the table, I could feel my face become flushed and the tears well up in my eyes. Maybe I wasn't tough enough for this place. Perhaps I should have never left my comfort zone and entered a world where life and death are literal components of every single shift. Before I could say a word, my charge nurse approached me and told me to stop. She could see what I wasn't saying out loud written all over my face, and she halted me dead in my tracks.

"This is not your fault. Sometimes these things happen. We did everything possible, but sometimes that isn't enough. We can't save every patient, every time."

She insisted that I take a walk – grab a cup of coffee, take a breather, maybe even go cry in a bathroom – but refused to allow me to take credit for such a devastating loss.

Every nurse was once a new nurse, and every nurse has a story similar to my own: one that forced him or her to question why she even decided to enter the profession in the first place. I don't care if you work in the most cheerful newborn nursery or the most sick-as-hell ICU in the place: really, really bad things are going to happen, and sometimes you'll be the one that carries the weight of it all. Never once during nursing school did anyone explain to me what emotions run through your head after bagging your first body. Nor did any instructor prepare me for blood-curdling screams and tear-streaked faces of loved ones who are devastated by an unexpected end. Hitting the "start" button on a morphine drip – one that ultimately would stop my patient's respirations and eventually their heart? There's no chapter or quiz to cover that one, either.

Learning all of the nursing basics is hard enough: the tenets of patient safety, medication administration, knowing when to contact a physician (and how) are just the tip of the newbie iceberg. Now add traumas and codes and emergency surgeries into the mix – well, no wonder we question what the hell we are doing so much of the time! The most critical lesson I've learned that I hope to pass on is this: it never gets easier. You simply learn how to deal with the really bad days in a variety of ways. Hopefully these methods – part defense mechanism, part cheap therapy – are enough to send you to bed after a really awful day, and allow you to wake up hopeful to return to work the next.

Laugh It Up

For nurses across the spectrum, laughter isn't the best medicine: Ativan is. Laughter, though, that holds a solid number two spot. If you want to make it through crawling and learn to walk the nurse walk, you're going to need a sense of humor to do it. Humor is the crutch with which beaten down nurses limp through a bad shift, and it's the icing on the cake of a good one. If nursing school wasn't enough to give you the giggles, the demented, dark, and slapstick antics that earn laughs at work will have you rolling on the floor. The phrase, "I laugh to keep from crying?" That surely must have been thought up with nurses in mind.

Deep in the gallows, you'll find a long line of nurses waiting to blurt out their royally messed up thoughts. As a newer nurse, I quickly discovered that the only way I could survive the literal life or death scenarios that come with managing serial emergencies is through humor. Laughter – though sometimes considered to be inappropriate, uncomfortable, or off-color – is a necessary means for newbie nurse survival. You're going to walk into work one day and realize that Rome is burning: you're short-staffed; the patients are confused and climbing out of bed; every test, procedure, or admission that can go wrong, does. This is simply the reality of nursing in general, especially in a hospital setting – some days just flat-out suck. The best weapon in your heavy-artillery nurse arsenal during these trying shifts is the ability to laugh despite it all.

Whether it's a gentle roasting from your fellow colleagues or a patient who makes you laugh until your stomach aches, the melodious musical notes of laughter often decorate the sickest and saddest settings. It isn't that nurses are not insensitive to the needs of their patients, nor do we revel in the pain and suffering of others. Instead, when death and destruction are running rampant across a unit, sometimes the only saving grace is a wayward stare and a well-timed dick joke. I've had moments in my career when I've been judged for seeming too cheerful, coming across as too "happy" to fit into my ICU environment. Eventually those naysayers became aware of the fact that an upbeat demeanor didn't mean I wasn't observing, synthesizing, and feeling: rather, it was my method of containing it all. So if you need to laugh, for Pete's sake, laugh: make a joke; be silly; giggle if you must; find a way to let the emotional strain and physical stress project itself outward and not in. People are going to die. Patients are going to suffer. It's not a funny place. It's not always a happy ending. But how you deal with it? That's what helps we nurses find joy in the good days, and survive the rough ones.

Cry It Out

Six weeks into my nursing orientation in the cardiothoracic ICU, I started to experience a roller coaster of emotions to make you realize you're human twice over. And yet a mere month and a half of excitement, adrenaline, confusion, concern, hopefulness, hopelessness, and faith that it all somehow matters paled in comparison to thirty-plus years of exhilarating and excruciating bedside experience contained within my own personal Socrates: my preceptor. When my primary mentor casually mentioned she had spoken on behalf of our team at a Moral Distress Committee meeting that would seek to improve end of life care in an intensive care setting, I was curious to hear what she had to say. In fact…curious is hardly a strong enough term: desperate is more like it.

What could a calm and collected, all-knowing and ever present ICU veteran have to say about living and dying after having been exposed to both ends of the spectrum and everything in between for three decades? The words she had written summarized exactly why this job is so damn cool and so painfully complicated in the exact same breath. As I read the introduction to her lecture during my introductory ICU nurse days – twice, because it had to really sink into my head – I felt a heightened sense of obligation to the patients under my care. Whether they should fight to live or die with dignity, it is the nurses caring for them that carry the brunt of the burden. Of course families suffer. Certainly physicians are concerned. Yet it is the nurse, whether tough as nails or still timid and learning, that bears witness to a patient's final breath. Sometimes, it's a peaceful transition; others, a tumultuous battle, but every time, meaningful in some way. Whether you're newly indoctrinated or have been saving lives for years, we can all benefit from the wisdom contained within someone who has truly woven the fabric of our nursing cloth.

My preceptor taught me one incredibly powerful thing about being a critical care nurse: there are going to be days when you need to cry, because it feels like the only right thing you've done all day. Whether it's feeling challenged by an ethical dilemma or being a part of a traumatic and dramatic no-holds-barred death, we as nurses are important, bright, and strong – but we're also scared, confused, and human. If only our patients and their families knew just how many tears we've shed on their account – be it privately in a long, hot shower or as a team in the middle of the nurse's station – they would never believe that we were the same men and women who battled death and disease just moments earlier. I'm not telling you that it's okay to sob uncontrollably onto your keyboard every shift – but some days…if you don't know them yet, you'll know them eventually – well, it's the only way to make it through another thirteen hour day.

When I first started as a nurse I was constantly confused by my own emotions – how the hell can I be expected to leave everything at the door, when I've connected with my patients and their families for hours? Days? Sometimes, even months? Often, my writing, doodling, and journaling is born of a shift where I feel particularly guilty about my patient's condition. It's not that I did anything to cause my patient to suffer from infection or instability or infirmity, but at times we all feel burdened by the glimmer of hope in the family members' eyes that no longer shines within any of the care providers. How is it possible to simply clock out and turn off the human side of yourself without questioning – could I have done more? Should I have done more? Is there any other way? I don't know. I'll never know. But one thing I'm certain of is that I'm not alone in how I feel from time to time – whether you're brand new to your role or have a lifetime of experience, sometimes you cannot *not* carry your patients with you.

When you don't see me, it doesn't mean you aren't on my mind. Often times I leave your side begrudgingly, at best. Perhaps I'm being forced to take five or grab a snack by a fellow nurse down in the trenches, that sees my jaw is tightened and my eyes, entranced. Maybe I'm rummaging through a compartment filled with medications to protect your body, ease your pain, calm your anxiety, or increase your dangerously low blood pressure. I might be double checking a policy for a procedure that I must conduct; recruiting a hand to help turn you, bathe you, or reposition you; or confirming with a physician what the plan is for your care.

When you don't see me, I am still there. I might be tied up with another patient or family member. Sometimes, if you're well enough to notice that I'm missing, I am being forced to dedicate my time and energy to another patient who is struggling in some way. There are moments in my world when hearts stop beating. Sometimes, lungs stop breathing. Kidneys fail and infections prevail and sometimes, 'alive' means just barely hanging on. I hope to keep you unaware of that shearing thread, but I promise: if you were in their shoes, I would hold it taut from end to end.

When you don't see me, I don't want to ignore your requests – I promise that I think of you while I'm caring for others. I cannot always offer you water to drink or a bite to eat because of reasons beyond my control. Not only am I here to assess your pain and your body and your vital signs, I must also make certain that every thing you do is safe. Call me a goody-two shoe, 'Nurse Ratched,' or overprotective: I won't budge on your well being, despite your complaints. With intensive care comes aggressive scrutiny. But your new room might not be ready. I've probably already paged your doctor. And I've called your family twice to ask them to bring your glasses. Please be patient with me – especially when you don't see me.

It's often as though I function with two brains: one dedicated to the task at hand, and another that concentrates on what is yet to be completed. My to-do list grows as the moments tick by, and suddenly thirteen hours have flown and I am down to the wire. There is so much that I wanted to do for you – so very much I wanted to give – yet the day has escaped me and I must concede to my relief. I try to take pride in my checklist, but many times feel failure all the same – one person can't do it all; can't fix it all; can't kiss boo-boos and make everything right. I'll be damned if I didn't wish that's the way it worked some days.

When the paperwork is finally finished, thanks to a push from a granola bar and stale cup of coffee, I swipe my badge but cannot quite 'clock out.' I lean against a rusted locker, fielding my belongings while I attempt to collect my thoughts. That's when the questions and queries begin.

When you don't see me, while I'm driving in my car – some days blaring the radio to block out the past, others riding in stillness to silently reflect – I carry you with me.

When you don't see me, stepping into my home, stripping out of the shift's worries and into my own – I carry you with me.

When you don't see me, questioning what happened and why; whether I could have done better to help you survive – I carry you with me.

When you don't see me, tear streaked and red, filled with pain for your family, children, and friends – I carry you with me.

I carry you with me, whether you know it or not, because while I want desperately to leave your story at the door, I can't help but hear the pages echo in my heart.

I carry you with me, as a trophy or a scar, because that experience forces me to power through the days when all I want to do is throw in my stethoscope and walk away. For scars often fade while trophies are proudly displayed; but sometimes the quietest moments and simplest interactions are the most often replayed.

> *When you don't see me, I am fighting for you.*
> *When you don't see me, I am rooting for you.*
> *When you don't see me, I am praying for you.*
> *And sometimes, when you don't see me,*
> *I am mourning for you.*

I carry you with me. I am your nurse. So when you don't see me, please know that I'm near. Your life is my responsibility – your livelihood, my pride. We carry you with us: on scribbled notes in pockets, through aching within worn bodies – forever in our minds.

Drink it Down (or Find a Hobby)

It doesn't matter if you've been a nurse for days or decades – this profession can start to get to you if you let it. You might leave your shift in a pissed-off, beyond-annoyed, anti-management huff, wondering why you even bother going to work if you don't have the resources required of the job. You may leave after getting into a spat with a nurse colleague or physician, feeling belittled or undermined in your practice. You might have the best shift of your life – the most epic save; the most adorable baby; the most inspirational patient may impact you in a way that will last you a lifetime. Or you might experience the worst shift of your career – you mess up and can't let it go; an ugly trauma; the loss of a child; the list, as a new nurse and beyond, is potentially endless.

So go out for a drink with the crew at eight o'clock in the morning. Write in a journal. Bake a cake. Go for a run. Plant a garden or go antiquing or lobby for local government. Find any way – do anything – that can allow you to divest yourself from all you've invested in your day. I don't care if that means eating ice cream in your pajamas while watching a Netflix marathon on your entire day off: you need to find a way to decompress, because if you don't, it damn near may destroy you.

You entered this profession understanding that stress was going to be intimately linked to the job you conduct every day. It's going to frustrate the hell out of you that most people don't understand this, and they never will. Your family is going to get pissed that you work the holidays, as if you choose to schedule yourself on the holly-est and jolliest days of the year. Your partner may seem clueless to your needs, because he or she can never quite grasp what is truly an "emergency" and what are just minor details. Your friends will find it "so cool" that you only work three shifts every week, completely unaware of your desperate need to reflect, recharge, and recalibrate during that precious time away from those hospital walls. And you will question so much of what you've done and where you are going. You will feel that nursing is your shadow and it follows you from the moment you wake up until you're fast asleep. Cut the cord. Separate the need to let your profession rule your life. Once you become a nurse, you can never *not* be one: I wholeheartedly believe this. However, maintaining passion for the profession and keeping yourself excited about going to work every day depends on your ability to distance yourself from the work you do during the appropriate moments. A well-rounded nurse is a happy one, and as a new nurse this may prove difficult at first – you will learn. Whether your "me time" takes place in a bar or a bookstore, permit your self to own it consistently and enjoy it with gusto. A nurse will always be who you are – simply remember that work will always be there, so cherish the times when you are not.

With that being said, nursing is a profession must be pursued with caution – it constantly ranks not only among the most stressful professions, but also the most dangerous as well. The unpredictable physical nature of the job coupled with the emphasis on ethical standards and patient satisfaction make for a complex breeding ground of emotions. Who are we expected to protect, and how, if we ourselves are not protected? When these factors are taken into consideration, it's no surprise that there exists what is considered a silent epidemic of substance abuse among nurses across all sectors of the profession. Alcohol, prescription pills, and illegal drugs are a real problem that plagues the profession, and while I cannot speak to specific percentages and numerical data, I can tell you that it probably happens more than you might expect. You may be sitting here thinking to yourself, "I can barely keep up with my job sober – how the hell could I function while impaired?" With enough stress, time, and excuses, anything is possible. The path toward self-medication is a slippery slope, and if you or someone you know is experiencing a problem with substance abuse, it's imperative that you seek out help immediately. Not only is it in the best interest of the patients charged with your care, it's a clear sign that you are dealing with stressors in a way that can be corrected, avoided, and managed – but you cannot do it alone. This is the part of the book where I hand out D.A.R.E. T-shirts and expect you to roll your eyes at me. I promise you: I'm not some holier than thou perfect nurse who exists without flaws. We are all human, and we are all allowed to err as such – but some mistakes should never be repeated, and once they are repeated consistently and uncontrollably, the disease of addiction must be considered. So enjoy yourself; live your life to the fullest; seek whatever pleasures bring you nurse joy – but if your actions become bigger than you are, it's time to look inward and find a healthy resource. Telling your boss might be painful, but inadvertently killing someone while you are under the influence? Well, that's something you may never bounce back from.

Honey, I'm Home!

Everyone is looking for that special someone: the eternal soul mate; the love of your life; the other half with whom you hope to grow old and gray. Everyday I wake up feeling blessed and thankful that I was able to find my amazing husband: he balances my crazy. He remains rooted to the ground while I fly into the clouds, and is always ready to catch me if I fall. And despite the fact that he doesn't understand any of my medical jargon, he always tries to keep up with my war stories. But it takes a genuine effort on both parts to make our priorities work. Baby nurses, you're going to be in for a rude awakening when you come to the realization that handling you during your initial foray into this profession will be no easy feat. Dating a nurse is not for the faint of heart: just ask my adoring husband, who dealt with me as a neurotic, overworked, underpaid nursing student, and chose to marry me anyway. There's a strange irony in the fact that you're going to need strong partner to balance you out. On the surface, it would seem that nurses are caregivers; fixers; sex-pot Mother Teresa's or strong and stable men with hearts of gold. But when it comes to relationships: well, we can be as complicated as that admission from the ED at three o'clock in the morning.

To know a nurse is to love a nurse, but perhaps loving a nurse isn't all it's cracked up to be. On the surface, we seem like the best possible romantic partners. No matter the gender, there are certain qualities that are attributed to nurses across the spectrum that make us seem not only highly "dateable," but even like bona fide marriage material. Whether it's an online dating profile or a friend of a friend, men and women alike seem drawn to the idea of dating someone who's professional premise centers on caring for others.

Smart. Compassionate. Kind. Free physical assessments. And that whole "naughty nurse thing?" It's a thing for a reason. In fact, there's even a psychological term for "an intense attraction to female nurses." If you believe that you know someone who suffers from a case of "threpterophilia," (which, I would imagine, can be an equally intense attraction to male nurses as well), it appears that you're not alone. So why are nurses such a hot commodity in the romantic sense? And can you handle the pressure whether you are dating someone new, or have an established committed partnership, in addition to your infinite workload and tremendous sense of responsibility? In a word: are nurses dateable?!

Well, I've got news for you: we're f*cking human. Contrary to what stereotypes may teach us, not every nurse makes a perfect mate. Most of us don't fit into the prescribed list of attributes that are so commonly applied to those in the profession. As a matter of fact, I've compiled a list of *actual* reasons to date a nurse, since you're probably feeling pretty down on yourself after that ass kicking you got at work today! Kissing boo-boos and caring for old people are all fine and dandy, but the real reasons nurses should feel like beloved and coveted romantic Gods and Goddesses include the ridiculous and slightly sarcastic list below:

1. **Our sense of adventure.** We don't shy away from anything new; crave adrenaline during even the most mundane times; and we will literally touch anything with a pair of gloves on.

2. **Our sick sense of humor.** It's dark. It's twisted. And it's absolutely hilarious. As a matter of fact, some of the things that come out of our mouths are so shocking that they might make others think twice about that whole "starched white cap" business. If you think your partner is into you now, just wait until you hear your hilarious story about that rash! (Wait…you mean most people don't find bodily fluids hilarious?!)

3. **Our ability to fight for what we believe in.** Whether it's advocating to protect our patients or defending the honor of our fellow nurses, we are passionate about what we want and need. There's a pretty good chance this translates into our personal lives as well.

4. **Our flexibility.** Physically and emotionally "bendy."

5. **Our sense of perspective.** When you work in an environment where the pendulum of life and death swings back and forth every shift, you learn to let the little things slide. Laundry not done or some dishes in the sink? Not the end of the world. Nobody died, right?

6. **We know how to start a party.** Nurses are notoriously good at happy hours and social engagements, even if the party doesn't start until 7:00am. We work hard, change lives, and make clinical decisions every day – don't be surprised if we're planning for a night on the town or a weekend getaway to balance our reality.

7. **We don't need you.** It's great to have a partner, but with so many opportunities to work in various nursing arenas, we often keep them around because we want them there. Though we don't earn

nearly as much as we should, we can find a path toward financial independence that allows us to maintain a comfortable lifestyle.

8. **Smart is sexy.** Did you know that the Bachelors of Science Nursing (BSN) degree has been chosen as the toughest degree among all the college degrees by the Guinness Book of World Records? Brainless is boring.

9. **We're excellent problem solvers.** We are faced with challenges in staffing, supplies, and circumstances every day in our careers. Much like MacGyver in a pair of scrubs, if you've got a problem to work through, odds are a nurse can help you navigate it. If we don't know the answer, we're pretty damn good at finding one. And if you don't know who "MacGyver" is, I've apparently just dated myself as older than I care to admit.

10. **We clean up nicely.** Don't be surprised to find nurses looking one way in our work uniform, and blowing people's mind once the scrubs come off. That is, of course, unless they prefer us that way. Unfortunately, if it were those tiny white dresses and fishnet stockings you're looking for…well, even if we could run a code blue in high heels, nurse friends, we probably wouldn't want to. Patient safety, after all, is tantamount.

Loving a nurse requires a partner who is secure, passionate, and willing to take on the challenge. We may seem ideal on the surface, but we can be quite a handful. Some days we will be on fire from our day, while others we'll crave silence and solitude. If your partner has what it takes to deal with the emotional ups and downs that come with dating a new nurse, I have no doubt that they'll get to enjoy your more intriguing qualities in the end. We love hard. We give a damn. But don't expect us to bend over backwards, coddle, or remain quiet. Suitors beware: there's so much more to nurses than sweethearts with stethoscopes. Pursue with caution. Choose wisely. Be with the one who allows you to remain quiet when the silence speaks volumes, and lets you pour your heart out when it needs to be cleansed.

Save the TV Drama
for Your Mama

We've all done it: watched an episode of *Grey's Anatomy* while we were in nursing school and thought to ourselves, "I can't wait to see the crazy shit that happens once I work in a hospital!" And no, I'm not referring to the patient scenarios and clinical situations. I'm talking horny surgeons, late-night trysts in supply closets, call-room antics, etcetera and etcetera. You can fill in the blank with whichever ridiculously outlandish Shonda Rhimes situation strikes your fancy, but I must warn you, newbies, of one very important reality: if you shit where you eat, you're not allowed to complain when your meal really stinks!

Since becoming a nurse, I've constantly had two questions asked of me by family members, friends, and even total strangers: 1) what kind of nurse are you; and 2) is your job just like *Grey's Anatomy*? Don't get me wrong: I love me some Meredith Grey, and I can't get enough of the McDreamy versus McSteamy debate – but the sort of shenanigans that happen on a television show simply don't occur in real life. First of all, I've never had a surgeon start my IV line or escort my patient to CT scan, but I'll leave that for another book. In addition to the totally ludicrous plot lines involving patients and their conditions, the show has established some pretty absurd expectations for nursing staff regarding romantic possibilities within the walls of a hospital. I'm not saying that there's no chance of you meeting a gorgeous doctor who will sweep you off of your feet and make you the world's happiest nurse – I'm just saying that there's a decent chance that your stunning doctor is happily married. I'm not saying that you aren't entitled to spicing up your shift with a little hanky-panky in the call room – I'm just saying that seven patients, three admissions, q2 hour Dilauded, and a family that wants to speak to your manager will probably leave little room for you to take a pee break let alone much else. I'm not saying that dating your colleagues or coworkers is forbidden or frowned upon – I'm just saying that the walls of a hospital are made of big ears and quiet whispers, and everyone else might be the first to know every gory detail before you do. I'm not saying that gossip and trash talk is a good thing – in fact, it's the absolute worst – but your actions can very well reflect upon your career if you choose to act carelessly. If at all possible, try to be the nurse who leads with an air of mystery – you've got enough dirty laundry in the patient linen bins: don't let the whole unit in on yours. And if dismiss my advice and throw caution to the wind? Well, for f*ck's sake, be sure to make your story a good one!

Med School Dropout

Toward the end of a busy-as-usual shift as a nurse of six months, recently off of orientation and toddling around the unit like an energetic puppy that occasionally still wets the carpet, I sat back in my computer chair and exclaimed to anyone who might be listening: "Thank goodness this day is over!" This comment led to an interesting response from a neurology resident who was still reviewing the day's workload with her attending. "You know," she said, in a manner that was far more filled with envy than resentment, "one of my best friends is a nurse in the Emergency Department, and he gets to work three days a week and make double my salary." In an effort to delicately counter her perspective, I smiled and responded with a laugh: "I literally got peed on today. Like, a person peed on me. So it's not always as glamorous as it seems."

She and her attending immediately agreed – they could never do what I do, and frankly, I could never do what they do, either. This resident described to me her thankless hours of clinical and research which have accumulated to over three hundred thousand dollars in debt and no job in sight that could ever pay it back. She seemed to love what she was doing, but she stated this without the same passion that she likely had as a fresh medical student who believed that she could change the world and make some serious bankroll. Her work-life balance, without a doubt, has been impacted by the decision to pursue her career, as evidenced by her description of the "lazy ex-fiancé" whose fingers were practically arthritic from playing video games all day while she learned about neurons and axons and dermatomes and the like. For all intents and purposes, it seemed as though she lived her life as a person who only occasionally leaves the hospital to perform vital life functions (like eating, or maybe even sleeping).

The fact remains: I've already encountered numerous medical residents who outwardly declare that they are overworked, underpaid, and have little to show for it. They often compare themselves to the staff nurses at the hospital who, thanks decent compensation and a pro-nursing management team, are probably more satisfied than many doctors. And yet when I pose the question (usually with a touch of jest), "So why didn't you become a nurse," the response is always the same: I could *never* do what you do. Sometimes the response is genuine, and is followed by a sentiment of gratitude for all that nurses endure for their patients. But most of the time, the response goes hand-in-hand with a wrinkled nose on the face of a physician who could never, ever, in a million years, ever do the gross shit we do.

And so I often do what any good nurse would do, and provide an example of something exceedingly nauseating that I've seen or done or touched (always with gloves on, thank you), just to make the point perfectly clear to the down-on-herself doctor: nurses don't do what we do for money. There are probably seven million easier ways to make a buck than being a nurse. We also don't do what we do for the cushy schedule, because lord knows that thirteen-hour shift is anything but easy, even if only three days/nights/weekends/holidays a week. And we are *certainly* not all medical school dropouts. If we wanted to become physicians, many of us could have. Our skill set and knowledge base grows with every day of clinical experience. While physicians are trained to diagnose and treat, it is often the nursing staff that determines a change in patient condition, both subtle and obvious (can anybody say "code-blue?"). And when something goes wrong for a patient, ranging from mildly inconvenient to horribly earth-shattering, it is the nurse who is yelled at; complained to; turned to; cried on; and yes, sometimes peed on.

It is during these moments – the ones that make nursing so damn difficult but so worthwhile – that we should take a millisecond to stop and think to ourselves, amid the mess and the madness: you could *never* do what I do is right. As a nurse, you're going to come across questions from countless patients, family members, and even physicians regarding why you opted into nursing and not another profession. The conversation will likely come from a place of adoration and respect for your knowledge and skill sets, yet might feel like a backhanded compliment depending on the circumstances. Our role as nurses is not a glamorous one; it's not an easy one; it's not a pristine and perfect package and it never will be. But my guess is, baby nurse, you probably didn't enter the nursing field without knowing how to get your hands a little dirty. Accept the compliment; remain gracious; and if you're like me, dish a little right back to the grossed out physician who looks like he's ready to drop on the floor after seeing your rectal tube explode.

PART IV

OH SHIT!

CAN I REALLY HANDLE THIS?
Movin' on Up

Given enough time in the profession, it seems to be generally noted that nurse leaders and upper management are two very different breeds of administration. Upper Management is not the enemy…but she's not exactly your old chum, either. It's kind of like that old college roommate you lost touch with: she went on to marry some filthy rich hedge fund banker and shows up at your house one day wearing $2,000 shoes. Yet despite her selective memory and judgmental attitude, everyone knows that she was right there with you chugging beers and cleaning puke back in the old dorm room. Upper Management tries hard to relate to your way of life, but she doesn't understand the Target clearance section and a six-dollar bottle of Cabernet the way you do – at least not anymore. She's always going to be your old roommate, and you have that in common, but now she's just…different. The thing that separates the managers from the real leaders, however, is the connection that the latter feel toward the nursing profession, and how it still resonates in their decisions. A nurse leader may not get down and dirty with bedside nursing any longer, but he or she remains in tune with what you are dealing with every single shift.

As nurses at every stage of your profession, you'll rely on those leaders – the nurses who happen to work in an administrative setting and not the other way around – to advocate for you in every step of your burgeoning career. From actually giving you your first opportunity in nursing to moving on to whatever chapter might come next, maintaining a connection with the leaders of your hospital is an excellent way to prove your transferrable skill sets cross over every arena of a hospital setting. Someday, you're going to need those leaders – the damn good ones; the ones who fight for the staff and the stuff; the ones who acknowledge how hard you work and the good you do; the ones who promote an open dialogue in the setting of learning instead of retribution and criticism – and eventually, with enough growth, you're going to *be* them. Despite the stereotypes that follow nursing administration and their apparent disconnect from being "deep in the trenches," every one of those managers, directors, Vice Presidents, and beyond were new nurses just like you once upon a time. Work in a fashion that is respectful of what they can offer you, but also remain vocal about your thoughts, beliefs, and concerns. True leaders will listen, learn, and incite change; anyone who doesn't is probably not worth working for. Remember that a hospital is a business, but our commodity has no price tag: safe and effective patient care cannot be sold at cost. Even when upper management may try to lean down, skim the fat, and save a buck, a bad-ass nurse manager is all it takes to say, "not my unit, not my nurses."

Holi-Dazed

Since you clearly knew what you were signing up for before embarking on your path to nurse-dom, I don't have to warn you about a feature of the job that is almost completely unavoidable: sharing holidays with your coworkers. Whether it's having a summer barbecue in the staff lounge in the heat of July, or feeling merry and bright with your team in the winter, you're going to have to get used to kissing your own family and friends goodbye at least some of the time. This topic always seems to be a point of contention for many nurses I know. The idea of leaving your own loved ones behind for the sake and safety of total strangers is a challenging one, yet whether it's your first day as a nurse or you've been working for years, the expectation is that a hospital isn't going to close down on account of turkey and football on Thanksgiving. If you work in an institution similar to my own, the holidays are paired off and staffed based on seniority preference. That can mean it takes a decade – literally – before you earn the privileges of having the shift off on your most anticipated holidays.

The flip side, however, is this: you are considered an *essential* employee. You are a fundamental component of our society, and because of your relative importance compared to, say, almost everyone else in the world, you are one of the select men and women who plays a role so pivotal that it must continue twenty-four hours a day, seven days a week. As a newer nurse you're likely to become frustrated by the nature of your schedule – night shift, weekends, holidays – you'll get a taste of every combination. You will absolutely miss out on cookouts and beach days in the summer, and ugly-whatever-sweater parties in the winter. You will undoubtedly be accused of bailing on your friends and their life-altering social engagement of the week. Your significant other will definitely have to defend the fact that they've not contrived an imaginary partner to discuss with mom and dad and wacky Aunt Sally around the holidays. You will certainly miss out on bridal showers and baby showers and, sometimes, literal showers on account of your ridiculous schedule. You will be an enigma to all who question how it's possible for someone who "only works three days a week" to be so busy all the time. The thing about it, my friend, is this: the others simply do not understand what you do. They truly cannot fathom the fact that we work "only three days a week," because those days are not only long but they are hard and stressful and require our minds to function at its maximum capacity. They cannot comprehend how we are so busy during our days off, yet they have no understanding of our overtime commitments, committee requirements, hospital engagements, and continuing education components. They cannot treat us like their "other" friends or family members because the others do not require literal respite from human contact after the very worst day. Because sometimes, it's so f*cking difficult to go out and grab a drink or have some dinner or catch a movie when you've got the blood of another human being on your hands. Despite the fact that it's not your fault they didn't make it, you're going to feel like it is.

So while they blame you and they question you, remember that they know not what you do. While they call your profession thankless, difficult, and question why they would make "poor little you" work under

108

such circumstances, remember that you earned your spot deep down in the trenches. While they ask why "it's always you" that must work on Memorial Day Weekend or on Football Sunday or during your cousin's uncle's boss's wedding, remember that not everyone can do what you do – that's why you must toss on your scrubs, wipe down your stethoscope, and handle it.

My perspective on working the holidays was completely rocked once I transferred to the intensive care unit. Suddenly it hit me: all of the meaning behind giving thanks; all of the buzz about hope and peace and joy; all of our freedoms, and how we take them for granted. It became clear to me that we – the Holiday Warriors – we were not unlucky to be working during life's precious occasions. Oh no...indeed, we are the fortunate ones.

We are the holiday warriors. The "tis-the-season" team. My fellow nurses – along with the nursing assistants, respiratory therapists, physical and occupational therapists, physicians, advanced practice providers and others – we are the Pilgrims of a brave new world. We are the holiday elves that push to place our patients on the good list – one that allows them to survive another wintry night and see another day. We are the whimsy workers in a winter wonderland that literally chill our patients with the intention of preserving their brains after cardiac arrest. We are the Turkey Day brigades who place and manage balloon pumps instead of watching balloons along Macy's Day Parade; who breathe life and circulate blood into the bodies of those who would surely give thanks if they could. Tryptophan is at the very bottom of the list of chemicals that concern us, for with emergency heart surgery we are enemies of sleep.

We are brown gravy warm and pumpkin spice sweet, ensuring that our patients and their families can celebrate a time of thanks within reason – given the circumstances in which they find themselves. Us nurses – on the floors; in the operating room; in the ED or the ICU, we feel the constant pressure: you're guests in our home, and we hope to provide you with exactly what you need to drift through the holidays into a brand new year. The reality is, some of our patients won't make it through the holidays. Some may barely survive the shift. Despite our best intentions; despite our strongest efforts; despite the advances that science and technology can offer: some will still die – leaving our elven spirits tarnished, our thankful hearts in pain.

So if you have the chance to spend this holiday season with your loved ones, soak in every moment – the colorful sights, the delicious smells, the sound of laughter that comes from satisfied bellies and full hearts. My family is always disappointed when I tell them that I'm scheduled to work my thirteen hour shift on the holiday, but I gently remind them the simple reality: *I signed up for this*. I entered this profession understanding that I would have to sacrifice my time around the holidays to take care of the infirmity of others. So when my alarm clock sounds early in the morning and I put on a fresh pair of scrubs, I look up to the sky and give thanks: I'm thankful for the opportunity to help save the lives of those who have seen the darkest of days. I'm thankful for cold turkey and all of the fixings that punctuate my lengthy to-do-list. I'm thankful for a team of coworkers who are more than just colleagues – but family of the most dysfunctional kind. And I'm thankful for the families who allow me to see what gratitude truly means, and how grand blessings can be counted in the smallest ways.

Tube feeds and turkey. Sepsis and stuffing. Code blues and "thank you's" and teamwork and tears. I am a holiday warrior – I am an ICU nurse. Even when my feet are sore and my belly is hungry – every holiday, every shift – my heart is full. Baby nurse, don't ever forget why you're essential. Without nurses, a hospital is just four walls; a heart is just an organ; and a holiday is just another shift.

An Empty Pot

Unless you're in the mattress business, a hospital bed is a horrible place to be. Now imagine receiving an education that focuses on every last thing that could go wrong with a human being; working in an environment where people with a slew of maladies and diseases surround you; and having yourself or a loved one end up requiring medical care. One of the implied functions of the nursing profession is becoming everyone and their mother's go-to source of professional advice. And while we must take every precaution to never ever practice outside of our scope and make diagnostic or prescriptive offerings unless legally capable of doing so, your family and friends will try to use you for free advice anyway. When a loved one falls ill, don't be surprised when you feel compelled to jump in and attempt to manhandle every aspect of their care. Whether your child requires antibiotics for a nagging infection or a parent has a serious health scare, brand new nurse or not, you're likely one of the most well-versed and medically literate resources available to them.

The interesting thing about becoming a nurse that there are some universal truths that seem to apply to every member of the profession across every spectrum: taking care of others before we care for ourselves seems to be one of those maxims. For starters, I acknowledge that this is a terrible way to live. There's a saying that goes, "One cannot pour from an empty pot," or some shit. I came across this pearl of wisdom beneath an illustration of an empty coffee pot pouring diddly-squat into a mug. Full disclosure: this was a picture on Pinterest. Fuller disclosure: I was searching how to cook the perfect filet mignon without burning a thirty-five dollar cut of steak, so I wasn't really paying *that* much attention. Fullest disclosure: I totally burned the steak. But in scrolling down the page, something about this image stuck with me enough to mention it in my first book...so to whoever created that Pin, I thank you for your Pinspiration.

*** *Goes to Starbucks for coffee. Suddenly whatever train of thought Sonja had was derailed and can only be repaired with caffeine.* ***

Like I was saying, as nurses we have a tendency to stretch ourselves pretty thin – this becomes especially true when a loved one becomes injured, ill, or incapacitated. We seem to take on the obligations that come in tandem with the circumstances. This can range from literal tasks such as doctor's appointments, testing, and hospital visits, and stretches its rope all the way to the top of Maslow's Hierarchy in offerings of emotional support and guidance. Our position in our families is often the rock: we are the strong ones; we are the capable ones; we have seen others suffer and know what should and could be done, and with enough experience, seem to understand when enough is enough. As a new nurse, you will soon be caught in a conundrum: while you feel as if you know nothing, those around you will look to you for your sage wisdom. You might go to work and feel totally clueless, and then come home to questions, concerns, and decisions that imply the total opposite. Take it from me: all it takes is one bad experience on the other side of that hospital curtain to make you realize what a patient and family member is looking for in a nurse. Whether you require an emergency appendectomy or have a sister in labor or sit with a best friend with an unexplained lump on her breast, each of these experiences will force you to balance your nurse side with your human side. You probably won't understand the difference until you're placed in a situation that shows you that being a nurse who is a family member or friend, is not the same thing as being a family member or friend who is a nurse.

My mother isn't my best friend – our connection is much weirder than that. We are akin to soul mates. She and I have some kind of sixth sense vibe that happens when one or the other has an issue – physical or emotional. Likewise, she always seems to know about the happy times and good news before I even disclose the details. She and my father came to the United States from the mythical land of Macedonia (Yes, it's a real country. Yes, it still exists. No, it's not the same thing as Mesopotamia, the ancient Parthian battleground.) shortly before I was born. They brought with them a staunch work ethic; advocacy for education for my sister and me; and the idea that their children would achieve a life of success that made their sacrifices worthwhile. Lo and behold, being a good human being doesn't negate the fact that bad things might happen. And so my nurse brain and my daughter brain embarked on an epic battle when what was presumed to be pneumonia turned out to be a mass on mom's right lung last summer. Thanks to conscientious and highly skilled compassionate care by world-class nurses, surgeons, and advanced practice team members, removal of her right lower lung and a four-day hospital stay eliminated the problem that was ultimately discovered to require no additional treatment. However...

In that moment – when time speeds up and stands still at once...when you receive a phone call that you'd recited in your mind a million different ways…when what you were hoping and praying and wishing to hear couldn't be further from the truth…that's when you know that being a nurse – though truly a blessing – can feel like a curse. (*I wrote and published the following on the Blog at The Huffington Post shortly after my mom's PET scan results – still unsure of what peaks and valleys we would be expected to conquer. There's a point to all of this emotionally gut-wrenching stuff: I promise.*)

The Phone Call

The strangest thing happens when people catch wind of horrible news. They suddenly become unable to appropriately verbalize what they are trying to say. There is a lot of I'm sorry; there is generally a look of absolute pity; and they almost always ask, "Are you okay?"

Of course I'm not okay. I'm at an absolute low point in my existence. In one three-minute phone call, I've been taken from a state of wonder and possibility to the horrendous reality of death and disease. But I won't tell you that. I won't say that aloud. When bad stuff happens, you're supposed to remain optimistic. You are supposed to say things like, "My mom is a fighter; she will get through this." You're supposed to welcome warm hugs and thoughtful messages. But you can't do those things forever, because you know too f*cking much. You find it nearly impossible to hope that maybe it was a false positive result, because you understand just how far technology has come. You can hardly listen as people ask you how she is dealing with it, because you know that she is pretending to be strong so that you don't worry. She even told you to make sure you eat your dinner, for Christ's sake, after handing off the news.

So you do what you did last time, when you were eighteen-years-old and without a worry in the world: you try to play the optimist. You smash the news into the corner of your brain and convince yourself, tear streaked in the locker room mirror, that you can work the rest of your shift because everything is going to be okay.

But it won't be okay. At least not the same way it was before. Because she's older now; and she's sicker now; and she made it perfectly clear in very plain language that if this thing on her lung is too far advanced, she's going to refuse treatment. So you smash her words into the corner of your skull and refuse to believe them. You'll be okay. It will be okay. I'm okay.

Putting on a Brave Face

I deliver the diagnosis, first to my very-pregnant sister, and then my husband. I make it through with total lack of affect. My voice cracks a little while I tell Joe the news, but recover enough to convince him (or maybe myself) that I'll get through the next three hours of work without any problem.

My pep talk to myself is total bullshit. I can sense it from deep down inside, I'm about to burst but I shouldn't. That's not my job. I'm the sensible one. I've got rose-colored lenses. I'm supposed to keep it all together while everyone around me falls apart. I woke up Friday morning and put on extra-dark eyeliner. It was a trick that I used in 2004 when I thought I was going to have a rough day. I wouldn't cry if my eyeliner were thick. Then everyone would know. Everyone would see how I really feel, what I was going through. I couldn't let that happen. Not again. But I'm a different person now than I was back then. I've gone through the best and worst days of my life. I've learned what it means to love unconditionally. I've seen lives hang in the balance, and I've helped them transition into the afterlife. I am not the same. I will never be the same.

So when I walked into the unit, pretending to be totally fine and capable of caring for two critical patients, I could feel that lie start to unravel. With one look at my best friend at work – she knew why I took a call during my busy shift, and from the look on her face, she knew the news before I could tell her. With one glance, I unraveled. My face was hot and my brain became dizzy and I could feel my knees buckle from under me. This time, I found out the news – but I was not alone. This time, I knew what to expect. This time, I was left with no surprises.

They hurried me away into an empty patient room and sat me down on a trashcan while I hyperventilated. My words were incomprehensible. I don't remember exactly what I was trying to say but I do know that it ended with the fact that I cannot do this again...

Three of my best friends stayed with me despite the chaos on the unit. They wiped my tears. They made me laugh. They assured me that we would do whatever possible to get through one day at a time. My boss came in and told me that she had covered my assignment, and she took me off of the schedule for Saturday. The funny thing about nurses is they don't know how not to nurse. I couldn't have been in a better or worse place at the time. They insisted that I not drive, and my husband picked me up after speeding from the office to get me.

Softening the Blow

"Hey baby... I'm so sorry... are you okay?"
I'm still not okay.

He brought me a dozen roses and two pounds of chocolate. He understands that nothing he says at this very moment is going to help me, so he holds my hand silently. We grab some food at a mediocre chain restaurant, and I order a margarita the size of my head. After two sips I realize that if smashing the news into the back of my brain doesn't help, neither will drinking it away. I proceed to have water with my french fries, and we make fun of the very-corporate general manager and how he is a classic television trope.

Joe brings me to the standalone department store across the street. We gently poke fun at everything from the clothes to the customers to the fact that a standalone department store even exists in 2015. We enter the appliance section and pick out a $4,000 refrigerator for our imaginary house, and then make fun of people who spend $4,000 on something as stupid as a refrigerator. We leave empty handed, and my headache starts to subside after laughing and wandering for an hour.

I call my mom when I get home. I lie and say that I just arrived from work. She doesn't know how I handled the news, and at this point, she doesn't have to. I understand that lying about how I feel is just as bad as her lying about she is, but I do it anyway. She tells me not to worry. She insists that I not change my life because of her – that I absolutely must lead my life and pursue what I was already planning. And then she reminds me, just before we hang up, that she told the doctor her wishes: if it's "bad," and there is not treatment that will help, she wants nothing to be done.

> *"I've raised my girls. I've lived my life. And honestly, baby, I'm just so damn tired of it all."*

I agree with her. I tell her we have lots of steps before that happens, and that we need more details before we can make a plan.

I'm Not Okay

I hang up, still wearing my scrubs, and start pacing around the living room. Joe asks me how she is doing, and I remain silent. I pace from the living room to the kitchen. I go to the bathroom and brush my teeth. Once I enter the bedroom, I can feel every emotion inside of me inflating, like a bubble that's inevitably going to burst. And then pop. I ruptured.

Wide open. Spilling out from the very depths of my being. It was volcanic, and I began melting. I dropped to the hard wooden floor in my underwear, bargaining with God. I begged him. I asked him why he would do this again, and why to her. I asked him to give me her struggle and her pain. I couldn't breathe. I could feel my breath shorten, and my gasps were labored. My husband ran into the room and threw himself around me. I covered him with snot and tears and expletives. He held on so tightly that I could feel his hands gripping into me for dear life. It was as though he was holding on so that I wouldn't escape myself any further. It was almost an hour before I quieted down. Before I could feel myself coming back into a rational and reasonable state again. Wherever I went in that very moment, it was not within myself. The old me had bled out, and now I was reborn. I was back to being myself, but a new and different version. I couldn't be the old me anymore. BC: before cancer – that's how I am going to have to exist.

Joe helped me to my feet and I stood in the bathroom: hot, red, stripped in every sense. I looked at how green my eyes appeared – they always had a catlike glow when I cried, accented by a glassy reddish-white periphery. I took shower that was too long and too hot for 11pm on a Friday in August. When I crawled into bed, the heaviness of the day weighed down upon my body. I closed my eyes and fell asleep instantly, not waking up until 10:45am the next day.

"Are you okay?"

I will never be okay. I will never be normal. I will never be the person I was before that day. There will be really great moments and unspeakably challenging ones, but I am not ever going to be okay. But really, who wants to be "just okay" anyway? Today I am feeling quietly concerned but calm. Yesterday I was motivated to overcome the challenge at hand. Tomorrow? Who knows? Every single day will be punctuated by a different emotion, a different version of the woman who I am.

Please don't be sorry. Please don't feel badly. And please don't ask me if I'm okay.

You cannot – I repeat, you cannot attempt to take on everything alone and expect to be the hero. It's not heroic – it's stupid. It's dangerous. It's unhealthy for your body and dangerous for your psyche. You're going to start off feeling like you can tackle anything that is thrown your way in this life – being a nurse very well might make you feel invincible. You'll think to yourself, "Well, shit – if I could survive a day like that, I can handle anything!" But whether a soft newbie nurse of a hardened veteran, you may not always be aware of just how much support you have while you're tackling patient care at work. Even on your most difficult shift, you have nurse colleagues, support staff, physicians and practitioners. You take on some of the hardest hitting clinical scenarios, to

124

be sure – I'm not attempting to discredit the amazing work you do, and the amount of knowledge you acquire. But you cannot be the same nurse off duty that you are while on the clock. You cannot be present as your wife delivers your firstborn child and focus on fetal heart monitors and APGAR scores. You cannot meet your best friend having chest pain in the emergency department and fixate on troponins and ST elevations. And you cannot bring your mother for major lung surgery and not allow yourself to be her child first, and her healthcare provider second. I speak to you not as some distant narrator in a how-to survival guide for those new to nursing: I have 100% made these mistakes and lived with the consequences. Just because you think that you're strong enough to roll with the punches and take on the hits as they come, doesn't mean it's necessary. If you're an empty coffee pot, you've got nothing left to pour. If you don't take care of yourself first, you'll be hard pressed to do a decent job of caring for others – whether your own or complete strangers. Being a new nurse is one of the most stressful transitions you may ever experience in life. Unfortunately, just because you've taken on a tremendously challenging profession doesn't mean that life is going to treat you like a delicate flower in every other arena. Caregiver fatigue can crossover from your professional life into your private one – find someone to talk to when times are tough; find something to balance you when the days are rough; and work to discover meaning in it all when the nights are long. And if I can offer you the greatest insight into the littlest sentence? When your patients or their loved ones are slammed by a ton of bricks that is life-altering news, try to avoid asking them if they're okay. Take the educated guess that they aren't, and see how you can help out anyway.

OH SHIT!

I'M NOT A KID ANYMORE!
Jack of All Trades, Master of...Whatever

Imagine your future, nurse friend: once you've overcome learning where the dirty linen room and the CT scanner are located; once you've stopped holding onto the security blanket filled with notes and cheat sheets in tattered spiral notebook in the back pocket of your scrubs; once you've managed to make it through a code blue or two without crawling beneath the bed or jumping out of a window. Your future is bright, kid! What will you make of it?

This seems to be the natural progression of the profession these days – the question of asking nurses, some even fresh out of their graduation caps, what's next. I graduated from nursing school with professors nipping at my heels to apply to graduate school and pursue an advanced practice degree immediately. Everyone is different, and some people feel more prepared to embark on the world of increased autonomy and added clinical skill-sets than others. To be perfectly honest, when I graduated with my BSN I didn't know what the hell I wanted to do. I was quite certain that cardiac surgery got me all hot and bothered during nursing school, and I set my mind on weaseling my way into the unit as soon as possible. My experience in the intensive care unit has exposed me to a world of opportunities and interesting scenarios that confused me even more – could I see myself providing sedation as a CRNA? Would I expand my practice and treat the whole realm of lifespan as a family nurse practitioner? Or could I stay at the bedside, improving my clinical capacity and critical thinking skills while working a decent schedule while making a good salary? Maybe I could even nix it all and write books in coffee shops!

My answer is simple: I have no simple answer. In the past year or so, I have applied to, interviewed for, was accepted into, and turned down two of the top nurse anesthesia programs in the country. I was admitted into and deferred a Doctorate in Nursing Practice leadership program. From there I was admitted to and declined an Acute Care Nurse Practitioner program...not once, but twice. Most recently, after much deliberation, financial planning, meditation, pro-con listing, crowd sourcing, and internal reflection, I deferred a dual degree program that has nothing to do with nursing at all: at least, not directly. I thought that attaining a Master of Public Health and Master of Business Administration could some how help me to kick ass and take names on a more global scale. Instead...writing books in coffee shops it is! My indecision has little do to with a lack of direction or a tendency toward fickleness – although I am a tremendously picky eater; have trouble sitting still; and require creative pursuits to keep my hippie-dippy soul content. Instead, my troubles began when I started to listen to the opinions of others instead of searching within myself for an answer. Many pegged me with qualities that could excel in a nursing leadership position – honestly, my background in Corporate America probably helped that reputation to develop, but I wasn't quite ready to step out of the bedside ball field and onto the sidelines. Once I transitioned from an ICU nurse infant into to less of a dependent blob and more of a functional albeit angsty team tween-ager, the prospect of anesthesia piqued my curiosity. I listened to others who seemed to paint a picture of a financially lucrative field that allowed for reasonable work-life balance and the capacity to remain clinically relevant. All of this is very true! But...after my mom's cancer scare, I started to question my own motives in that direction. You see I really, genuinely like human beings. I enjoy interacting with patients, family members, and colleagues and peers. Would I – as a socially capable and easily bored type-A nerd – feel boxed into the field without room to spread my nursey wings? Would I attend school for three years full-time; quit my job; dedicate every iota of my being to an education in anesthesia; and then wake up one day, as I had in my previous career, confined by a paycheck but not engaged in the work I am doing? That fear resonated with me – and as I mentioned earlier, your own self-awareness is crucial in making these major life decisions!

Ultimately, I came to the conclusion that I would be happier, more fulfilled, and by proxy, more successful if I allowed myself to practice in a capacity where I could remain challenged, stimulated, engaged, and maintain an outlet. And so for now, I choose nothing. I'm allowing the universe to guide me to whatever may be next, and saving some lives while I do it. In addition to really, genuinely loving my job, I also love the idea of creating change in this profession in a more broad-strokes way. As an...um, Master of none...I can remain at the forefront of my practice while having the time and energy to devote to the other spokes on my life wheel – family; friends; intellectual pursuits; personal growth; and naturally, writing.

As my journey toward academic advancement continues to evolve, I want to remind you that an advanced practice degree is not the end-all, be-all of the nursing profession. You are more than encouraged to remain at the bedside and practice as an RN or LPN for the entirety of your career, and you can do so in a fashion that hopefully affords you a lifestyle that keeps you comfortable and happy. As the healthcare model shifts and legislation from state to state continues to change, the scope of practice of advanced practice nurses continues to be carved out and polished down. The field is relatively young, and so much gray area exists between family and acute care nurse practitioner roles, for instance, or the role of a CRNA versus a medical anesthesiologist. If your plan, like mine, is to eventually and inevitably teach someday down the road, you must consider the cost/benefit between obtaining a Masters or a Doctorate or a PhD. The profession is desperate for nurses who are highly skilled and educated to train the next cohort of new nurses in the future, and there are statewide and national incentive programs to help fund the education of qualified candidates.

Before you walk into your unit on your first shift and convince yourself that you need to escape the bedside with an advanced practice degree, keep in mind the logistics required of every move you make. Graduate school isn't cheap. It's going to cost you a pretty penny to embark on these pursuits, and while many hospitals offer tuition assistance programs, it hardly foots the entire bill. If you intend to work while in school, remember that it may take you longer to complete your course of studies, and you should pay courtesy to your managers in pre-planning your class schedule, required clinical days, etcetera. Further, if you take on the option of attending school full-time and working only per diem or not at all, this can be a major lifestyle change for you. If you've finally graduated with your nursing degree and started earning a salary – I don't care how much money you are making, some money is better than nothing at all – it can be challenging to return to the life of a lowly broke student. Finally, keep in mind that while nursing continues to evolve and push for advanced education requirements down the road – just take a look at the Institute of Medicine's report entitled "The Future of Nursing" for all of the gory details – there is potential for markets to become inundated with graduate-prepared nurses. If salary isn't a concern for you, and your heart is set on advancing your practice, then this may not worry you. If you reside in an area where nursing salaries run above the national average, however, you may be shell-shocked when you find that your entry-level advanced practice nursing salary is less than you made at the bedside as an RN or LPN. More letters don't necessarily mean more numbers. Though I believe the cost of education is well worth the return on your own growth as an investment, it may not always mean this growth is reflected in your wallet.

If you're a baby nurse and already itching to move onto the next step, your best bet is to shadow a CRNA in the operating room or follow an APN in the office or put a bug in the ear of an admissions counselor at a local university before taking the plunge. Advanced education can one of the most challenging and rewarding components of your career – but sometimes the only thing harder than being a new nurse is being a new nurse with a graduate degree, a butt load of debt, and minimal clinical experience as a frame of reference for what the hell you're doing. If you're planning on becoming a nurse midwife, you should probably make sure you don't pass out in a delivery room. If you want to become a family nurse practitioner, you should probably be certain that you can vibe with children and octogenarians alike. And if you're planning to become a nurse anesthetist, you should probably make sure you could pronounce the word "anesthetist." Happy trails, baby nurse! Whatever you choose to do, do it with passion; do it because you care; and if you're doing it for the dollar signs, you should probably try cooking meth or pole-dancing first – it's an awful lot easier!

The Great Escape

I can only offer you so much guidance, insight, and evidence of the stupid shit I've done to try to convince you that nursing is a life-changing profession that is as dynamic and challenging as it is rewarding. But as convincing as I might be, I can't force you to love your career. As someone who Houdini-ed my way out of a corporate career a few years ago, I can assure you that you aren't the first to opt out of what you thought you wanted: you certainly won't be the last. If you find yourself waking up and feeling miserable more often than not; if you feel such crippling fear and severe anxiety while you're at work that you're stalled to the point of inaction; if you feel such deep regret in your decision to pursue a career in nursing that you're plagued by resentment instead of pride; there's a very good chance that working at the bedside is not the place for you. What's far worse than feeling disdain or distress in your workplace, is feeling disinterested or disconnected entirely. This dissociated state of practice can set you up for the type of distractions that border on dangerous patient care. And since it is our moral and ethical obligation to do no harm to those charged with our care, a nurse at any point in her career – from a fresh green novice to expert level – must have the awareness of self to recognize when enough is enough.

If the flame fizzles out and you go to work for the paycheck and not the experience, you're setting yourself up for unconscionable mistakes and egregious infractions. I'm not implying that you need to wear pom-poms and cheer your way through every single shift – frankly, that's not only unrealistic, it can be super f*cking annoying. What you must consider, however, from your first foray into nursing and as your career progresses, is why you chose to become a nurse, and what you're doing to fan that fire. You're not going to be satisfied with 100% of your job 100% of the time – but you should, at least, feel invested in the work you do most of the time. Although you might ebb and flow between good shifts and difficult ones, you need to start paying attention when the tide hasn't shifted, and you feel like you're drowning. Some people might experience this at the onset of careers; others may go their entire professional life without enduring this struggle. What is crucially important in your professional practice is that you constantly assess, evaluate, and reevaluate where you stand, and what changes you can make to recalibrate as needed.

If you go through every decade of your professional life without a single second thought and never once feel discouraged, second-guess your decision, or waver in your position – congratulations! You're a talented and amazing super awesome mega-nurse! You're also lying to yourself. You're ignoring your emotions and, I'm not a betting gal, but sometimes I live dangerously – I would bet that your own self-awareness is being masked, compartmentalized, or tucked away among other elements of your life. Perhaps you're busy planning a wedding; starting a family; buying a home; taking care of a loved one; managing health issues; running an ostrich farm; etcetera, etcetera. We exist at the center of a wheel, and the spokes of our personal wheel change as we grow and evolve. Your nursing career isn't the entire wheel, but its position on your wheel can either help it to run smoothly, or will leave you at a halt. We as

134

practitioners don't exist in a vacuum, and as a new nurse you can barely imagine the multitude of stressful human interactions that will barrel into you throughout your career. You're going to be pummeled with physical exhaustion; emotional strain; societal barriers; financial uncertainties; literal matters of life and death – all of this while you're on the clock. It's okay to come to a point where you've handled all you can, and you choose to say you've had enough.

The bright side – if you ever do choose to leave the bedside and attempt another path in nursing, or even start a new career entirely – is that the world is filled with so many wonderful options and opportunities. A degree in nursing affords you multiple arenas in which you can utilize your expertise, none of which require you to work in direct patient care. In addition to home care, long term care, and managerial roles, such opportunities as case management, community health and epidemiology, insurance management, legal nurse consulting, pharmaceutical and medical sales, and teaching can permit you to expand the depth and breadth of practice away from the bedside. You can opt to work in a physician's office, a surgical center, an urgent, care, and other facilities where you can still work with patients while maintaining a work-life balance. Further, with the technological advances and push toward tele-medicine and remote healthcare offerings, there are only more opportunities coming down the pike in the years to come.

And if you've given it all you could and decide, nursing be damned...so be it. Take a chance. Step outside of the box. Explore a career that piques your interests, enriches your livelihood, and fans that flame. Just don't be surprised if – despite choosing to be a lawyer or a banker or a painter or a barista – you come to find that even while you're not working as a nurse, you can never *not* be one anyway.

Oh Shit!
Moments

I've had quite an impressive series of "Oh Shit!" moments in my nursing career, and I'm certain that I've got a bright future ahead filled with expletives and face-palms. The fact of the matter remains: whether you've been in this profession for thirty seconds or thirty years, there will come a time when you screw something up. It might be a faux pas that makes the whole team roast you for months, or – hopefully not, but potentially – a major violation of practice or protocol. I can tell you first hand that so many potential "Oh Shit!" moments will creep into your practice on the regular – your job is to catch them before it's too late, or before they impact your patient in some untoward way. Sometimes, though, "Oh Shit!" moments are what keep us sane where we work, because they give those in the trenches with us a good hard laugh. The following list – by no means inclusive – goes to show you just a few of the moments that have had me mouthing "WTF" over and over again, or perhaps left me in a fit of laughter that could only be contained by clocking out and leaving the hospital.

Oh Shit! I helped my incontinent patient out of bed to the chair while working on the floor, and naturally I made the rookie mistake of giving IV Lasix after pulling out his urine catheter. As the nursing assistant and I strapped him in to the partial-support standing lift, the wheel became stuck under the bed. Naturally, as I bent down to release the obstruction, my patient started to pee mid-air. Not knowing what to do, I grabbed an absorbent pad from the bed and tried to makeshift a diaper. Fortunately for the cardiologist – and unfortunately for me – my patient responded quite nicely to the diuretic. Before we could lower him onto the chair, I felt a warm stream of urine all over my arm. And in that very moment – I experienced one of the few pangs of regret about leaving my corporate job. Because while there were moments where I felt that I was being figuratively shit on in my media career, I was never literally peed on.

Oh Shit! I once transferred my elderly female patient to her bed in the step-down unit after cardiac surgery. She was five feet tall soaking wet, a peanut physically – but this staunch Catholic Hispanic grandmother of ten put me in my place. We wheeled up to her double room, which happened to house a male roommate. Due to the nature of our step-down beds, there were certain circumstances where mixed-gender rooms did, indeed, occur for short periods of time. It wasn't preferred or ideal, but it did sometimes occur. I had a very busy morning and was planning to admit a fresh post-op case, so without thinking to call up and check on the room I wheeled my spitfire patient upstairs. As soon as we pulled into the room, she took notice of her male suitemate, and proceeded to call me numerous unsavory phrases in Spanish. I thought to myself, *"Self, you've studied Spanish for all of high school and college: you should speak to your patient and reason with her!"* After I eked one sentence out, my patient grabbed the stethoscope wrapped around my neck and showed me who the real boss was in the matter. After getting a good whack or two in, another nurse and I were able to calm her down enough to sit back down in a wheelchair in the hallway until we could stat clean, move patients, and make a new bed for her elsewhere. Sometimes your patients are like paper cuts: the smallest ones can cause you the most pain!

Oh Shit! I had a habit of coming to work thirty minutes before my shift as a baby nurse to review my patient assignment, ponder my telemetry strips, and take a few deep breaths before diving into my day. One particular winter morning, I was reviewing labs when I heard one of the bed exit alarms sound. Another nurse and I rushed over to the patient room, who was apparently a multiple attempted-escape offender awaiting a bed nearer the nurse's station. Despite being a bilateral amputee, the patient had something of an ornery personality and didn't take kindly to the requests of nursing staff. As we hauled-ass into the room, assuming we would need the manpower to keep the patient from fleeing his bed, we caught him, quite literally, red-handed. Though the patient wasn't trying to leave his bed, he had been conducting a horizontal handshake with such gusto that he triggered the bed exit alarm. You could imagine my face – a new nurse, young, blonde, assuming the best in humanity – as I watched a patient with no legs whack off in front of me. And what makes it even more of an "Oh Shit!" moment? He didn't even stop when the night shift nurse and I caught him! On the contrary, with a grin and a laugh, he kept on trucking!

Oh. Shit. Is. Right. Nobody died in these situations, except maybe my dignity. And trust me when I tell you I could write an entire book about patient comments, awkward scenarios, and oopsie-daisy missteps made by my nurse buddies and me over the years. As a newbie, you're going to encounter the best and worst of humanity every single day. You can try your very best to approach the situation with grace and austerity, but let's face it: some stuff is way too absurd to not question if you're at work or being punked by Ashton Kutcher. So when "Oh Shit!" moments come your way, embrace them: they happen to the very best of us. Once the shift is over and the day is done, you may think back on those times as some of the most memorable moments in your nursing career…and an occasional few that you wish you could forget!

Big Girl (and Guy) Panties

Stretch your brain cells and think back to the history of this storied profession. Florence Nightingale fought for sanitation, cleanliness, and anti-infective practices before the germ microbe was even discovered! Talk about a nursing assessment ahead of its time: the woman was able to observe and perceive trends in patient conditions through visual means, and institute changes in practices and protocols that extended beyond countries and generations. The woman left her cushy and comfortable life to go serve as the first nurse manager during the Crimean War, and sent her work to India in hopes of decreasing infection and death rates among the British army. And us? We tweet.

My point is not that we should all suck it up and deal with unsafe work conditions, short staffing, or minimal resources: not in the very least! As a matter of fact, my insinuation is that as a new nurse, you're might feel like you've got the short end of the stick much of the time. You may believe that you're punished for being new based on the nature of your assignment, or you'll assume that you are being brandished a failure for reasons like stupidity or ineptitude instead of the actual reason: a legitimate lack of experience. It is impossible to know what the hell to do, if you do not know what the hell you are doing. I think that was Plato or something.

Whether you're a nurse who is new in general or new to a unit, a device, a procedure, or a practice, there will be moments when the frustration that sets in from not knowing or understanding something might make you feel inferior. Guess what? Everybody gets it. Everybody feels this way. Everybody goes through a moment of entitled brattiness that leaves you feeling "woe is me" about the circumstances of your job. My suggestion is that you allow yourself some time to wallow in the misery of your nursing existence, and then put on your big girl (or guy) panties and get the f*ck over it. Just climb out of the hole of self-pity in which you've fallen, dust off your scrubs, and get back to the task at hand. There is a distinct difference between drowning at work and needing assistance to help you safely navigate the waters of your stormy unit, and just being a whiney little turd. I've been there. I've seen both sides of the spectrum. I've felt annoyed, frustrated, and taken advantage of by a crappy assignment or a heavy pair or a game plan that required me feeling like the unit's personal bitch. I've also done my best to bend over and take it when needed, because sometimes that's the nature of the work: shit happens. Patients crash. Stable patients code and shaky patients get better. One of the best pieces of advice I was ever handed given the circumstances is to work like hell to front load your shift with all of the must-handle tasks that need to be done, so that you can safely and efficiently develop strategy C when plans A and B crumble before your eyes.

Being a team player is one of those traits that are highly regarded among your peers, mostly because nobody wants to listen to somebody bitch and moan about the same problem constantly. There is always a time, place, or circumstance when the fate of your nursing destiny and how your shift might play out is written on the bed board and you just know it's going to be a challenging day. Sometimes, it's okay to discuss with the nurse in charge or your unit manager if you believe that you are truly being punished or made to take an inappropriate assignment routinely. Alternatively, it is totally okay to speak up if you believe that a patient assignment is unsafe or beyond the scope of your current nurse capabilities. I tried to play that card the first time I was assigned a patient with an open chest. The head nurse, wouldn't ya know it – she thought through the assignment before sticking me in the patient room willy-nilly. With just over six months of ICU experience, she sandwiched me between two senior nurses who were encouraged to keep an eye on me, assist with any procedures, and help to clean any diarrhea that might have seeped through my scrub pants. I survived; the patient survived; my bookends to my veteran nurse sandwich? Just barely, but they made it, too.

You're going to have so many days as a new nurse that make you want to play the victim. You'll feel like everyone around you is sitting around sipping on coffee and talking about reality television shows while you bust your hump just to stay afloat. You're going to wonder why you stay late shift after shift, and everyone else manages to clock out on time, every time. You're going to incorrectly gather all of these pieces of evidence to conclude that you're being treated worse than the rest, and you'll hit a point when you finally speak up about it. I cannot stress to you enough the importance of maintaining a diplomatic approach and deferring to reason and logic over emotion when this time comes. Whining comes with consequences. Complaining, perhaps even more so. And I'm not referring to a punitive assignment or lack of help from others: a victim mentality in nursing is something that we as professionals have worked so hard to overcome. If we demand the respect and playing field of physicians and colleagues, we cannot be the first to moan and groan and whine and give up when the going gets too tough. And I don't even mean sick as shit, complicated, crazy crashing patient: I mean when we are asked to remain flexible or adaptable or take one for the team as a temporary fix. So baby nurse, do yourself a favor and maintain a sense of fluidity early in your practice or process, and allow it to carry you through your career. Stand up for yourself when needed, but also maintain enough of an open mind and sense of understanding that the odds that you're being sought out, bullied, or intentionally punished is less than likely. And if, for some reason, this is the practice of your current place of employment, use what you've learned about maintaining respect and dignity for all colleagues – from the top of the totem pole to the newbie base bottom – and work to inflect change upon the status quo. So go home after an especially bad day, peel off your scrubs, and drop your big nurse panties into the wash. You'll need to wear them again tomorrow, hopefully with a smile on your face and a challenge on your agenda.

Magic 8 Ball Into the Future

I went to a psychic on the boardwalk of the Jersey Shore during my junior year of high school. I paid five bucks to have my palm read by a woman with a bad perm job and a lazy eye – the side eye proved to me that she was legit! The thing about the psychic was that she gave me a reading that was equal parts confusing and creepy as it was spot-on. She told me I was going to become a super model, which at the time felt like the most realistic piece of information for a shallow blonde teenager with an aggressive spray tan and five-inch wedge-heels. Later that afternoon, I was approached by a modeling agency on the boardwalk that swore I had what it took to become a star! I should have probably assumed at the time that a psychic that cost less than a Happy Meal and the shady modeling agent were working in cahoots to prey on typical annoying teenagers, but instead I took it as proof that this woman could predict and plan the future. Oddly enough, when I looked back on a journal filled with her statements and visions a few years later, many of them hit very close to home. I've given up on the super model thing, however, since nursing is a far more exciting and glamorous profession.

Fast forward to my first day in nursing school eight years later. The anti-glam. The opposite of glitz, glitter, and worldwide fame. I had changed so much in a few years, thanks to my own personal journey, that there was no way even I could predict what was to come in the next few months, let alone years in advance of my future. Plan though you may, my nursey friend, sometimes life is going to veer along a course that takes you down an entirely different path than you'd imagined. My realization is that the future of nursing is exceedingly challenging to speculate. With every year comes a new crop of baby nurses; with every decade arrives a new technology or advancement; and in single lifetime a nurse can work in a profession that started one way and morphed into something entirely different.

The future of nursing, no doubt, is an exciting one. It's dynamic. It will be evolving with every shift in hospital systems and change in government policy. Our role as nurses is one that has been defined, revised, and redefined in countless ways over the past one hundred or so years, and given the infancy of the profession relative to others, some growing pains are to be expected. If you're on the precipice of entering the field, you may hear a confusing mix of reviews regarding the nature of the business. Some will tell you that it's not the way it used to be – well, no shit, Sherlock! – and will harp upon the glory days of a classy and distinguished group of mostly women who gave the bed baths the correct way (and without gloves, too)! Others will question your stupidity: why the hell would you choose to be a nurse? They will insist you should have entered finance or become a computer programmer or something, because that's where the real money is after graduating. Still more may assume that you're just like the "rest of them," and that you'll obtain just enough post-graduation experience to build your resume and move up or move out, depending on who is defining the move. Then there will be a few – and pay attention to these nurses, you're going to need them – who will speak fondly of the profession. There will be a few who have had the courage and critical thinking to embrace the changes and roll with the professional punches. There will be a few who, while they agree there is much room for improvement in the role, believe in the hard work and advocacy that they conduct every single day. There will be a few who are just the right combination of real and ideal; who understand the writing on the wall but hope to flip the script; who see the future advances of our profession as something that is different but not necessarily a bad thing. So pick these brains. Ask questions. Listen intently. Do not dismiss this myriad of voices – the good and the bad, the naysayers and the cheerleaders, because each sound helps to form a symphony that will serve as the soundtrack to your career. Will you go home at night and hear The Sound of Music? Or is it the theme some from Jaws? Do you hear a grand overture? Or is it the jagged cacophony of a horror film?

The future of nursing depends on you. What *you* bring into this profession will dictate whether others choose to remain a part of it, or damn the field to hell. Create a tune, every shift – every day – that inflects upon the ears of those around you. There are endless options in the nursing field. You can expand and grow into many directions in the profession, or you can opt to remain in one place and become a pillar of excellence in that role. But I beg of you: as a former baby nurse turned pretty good nurse turned baby nurse again turned pretty good nurse with lots of potential turned baby graduate school applicant extraordinaire turned baby author turned maybe future pretty good author, I implore you – *do not become an asshole*. Do not fall into the trap that has plagued this profession for decades on end. Do not do unto others as others have done unto you, because you believe it's a rite of passage or a pissing contest or a way to stake your position of superiority. Someday you are going to be one of the very many voices that create a song in the mind of someone new to what you do: leave that man or woman with harmony instead of horror. I truly believe that nursing is a profession that is not called upon to many. I believe that somehow we are led to a place where we take on the ailments and emotions of total strangers because we in some way feel compelled to help them through some of the best and worst days of their existence. I believe that nurses are human, and that humans have good days and bad days; great qualities and shitty ones. I also believe, however, that nurses unfairly pick on one another given the stressful nature of the role, and we lack outlets to prevent this untoward behavior. Become the nurse that remains bigger than this behavior. Be a nurse that is better than what has been done to you or others you know. Rise above the bullshit. Call it like you see it. Protect other nurses with the same sense of safety and security you would want for your patient. Don't believe the hype that eating your young is an effective form of growing a thick skin: it's simply a scare tactic that can cause more harm to staff and patients alike than good. Retaliating against a bully by being one your self is a temporary fix. It doesn't correct the root cause of the issue at hand, and it's a temporary Band-Aid that will eventually loosen and fall off. In the future of nursing, it's your job to compose a symphony. Not everyone can be the lead in the orchestra, and not everyone can play the same instrument, but when it goes well, the team can gel together to play a beautiful tune. Conduct yourself in a manner that allows you to be either the alpha or the beta when the time calls for it. Stand without being called upon, and speak without shouting. Grow into your practice, and once you've advanced, help others to grow along with you. The world is full of drama. There's death and destruction, hardship and heartache anytime you open the paper or turn on the television. Our nursing community, like it or not, is a microcosm of this space. When you feel like making a negative headline, step back, take a breath, and remember that only the worst news makes the front page. If they're going to share the news anyway – well, give them something *revolutionary* to talk about!

Unapologetically a Nurse

And so now I leave you, my nubile nurse friend, hopefully encouraged and discouraged and then uplifted and kinda confused and sort of scared but still excited all the same about whatever the hell you've gotten yourself into, and how you're going to make it through the day. I refuse to tell you that you're going to get past the initial blow of this profession and that someday everything becomes easier – because it doesn't get easier. You could be a tried and true veteran in the nursing domain and you're still going to muddle through shifts that kick your ass. You're still going to care for patients who make you want to gouge yourself in the eyeballs with a number two pencil. You're still going to become hot and bothered and heated all over when something unfair or unfortunate or unforeseen happens. But eventually, the hard days grow fewer and the great moments start to snowball. Eventually, you're tougher and wiser but hopefully still as kind and compassionate as the day that you first started. Eventually, you start to investigate the complexity of those around you – patients and doctors and nurses alike – and you start to weave together themes and ideas about just the type of person who voluntarily enters this space, and what they seem to get out of it. Not everyone enters this profession believing that it is a calling – this I understand. Some nurses enter based on circumstance; financial or schedule issues; perhaps pressure from family or even your self. Maybe it was always the plan, and now you're in too deep. However, whether you work your entire career at the bedside, or walk away and leave it all for something totally new: I have no doubt that you, once a nurse, will have changed the life of another human being. You, once a nurse, will have helped to save a life. You, once a nurse, will have gracefully transitioned one. You, once a nurse, will have provided professional advice or compassionate care to family and friends. You, once a nurse, will have felt outraged by your lack of resources. But you, once a nurse, will manage to work anyway. You, once a nurse, will have felt slighted by management; felt cheated by your leaders; felt insulted by physicians; or felt attacked by your colleagues. And yet still you – once a nurse – will have fought like hell for the sake of those charged with your care…and with enough passion, will tweak this profession where it desperately needs fixing.

This profession is by no means a perfect one. I believe the only way that the role of nurses and nursing can advance is through recognizing the value in enriching others to grow and learn, instead of beating, hazing, and minimizing one another. We need to emphasize standing together so we do not fall apart. I believe that nursing will only remain a respected profession once we value veteran nurses as beacons of light and sources of wisdom, instead of working, straining, and stressing them into retirement or submission. I believe that management is not the enemy, but sometimes they should be reminded of where they once started. And I believe that we nurses are far more dynamic and complicated than media, television, and society has deemed us. We are not a singular layer of white shoes and pure souls. Nor do we swallow the bitter pills that we pass in our medication cups, hungry for revenge and retribution. We have so much to say. We have so much to teach. We have come so far; yet have so much farther to go. Thank you, baby nurse, for letting me voice my thoughts on a career that has changed me – I truly believe that I have been altered by what I do, see, and learn every day. Let us all work toward showing the world the depth and breadth of our profession – be it a calling or not. Regardless of whether we are happy or jaded. Regardless of whether we are new, green and rosy or burnt like toast and on the outs. We all have something to learn: even more do we have to share. And here I shall leave you…with a letter that I wrote to…well, basically *everyone* after an especially difficult day. I addressed it to those who mean something to my life and profession, but perhaps don't quite understand the plight of a professional nurse. I was new in the intensive care unit and struggling to get my bearings, yet learning more than I could have ever imagined all the same. And so this letter – one that I encourage you to share with the spokes that make up your own wheel – is a way to close the conversation that we've started in this book…one that, I hope, will continue in your professional practice. If you haven't already realized it, you will come to find that others don't always understand what we see and do every day: and that's okay. The best we can hope to do is educate them when appropriate; cut them some slack when needed; and advocate for our patients *and* one another every goddamn shift.

"Open Letter from a Nurse"

To My Other Half

I can only imagine how difficult it must be sharing your life with someone like me. I do my best to remain your truest friend and confidante in our relationship, but the biggest problem is this: I am a nurse. The day you married me, you devoted your life to someone who devotes herself to others. And while this quality is something that is often praised, I have no question that you must find it challenging to handle at times (unless, of course, you too are a nurse). You are patient and kind, and you work so hard to support me in my profession. The caveat, however, is that nursing is not simply a profession: once you become a nurse, you can never not be one. Every effort we make to separate our identities from our professions is rendered useless, because we remain at our very core nurses. And while we are commended and praised for all that we do, you, too should be commended for what you endure. I'm sorry for the days that I come home and dump my entire day on you before my keys even leave the door. I'm sorry for venting, and short of complaining, I apologize for making my greatest passion sound like something of a burden. For all of the countless times you smile at me and say "Hi honey! How was your day?" and I suddenly burst into tears, I'm sorry. Even more so, for the days when I greet you with silence, and I cannot collect my thoughts enough to create full sentences, I'm sorry. I thank you for listening to me when I throw medical jargon around and pretending like you understand. I thank you for laughing at what I consider to be funny, that most rational humans believe to be reviled. And I thank you for understanding, with nothing more than a glance...during those trying moments when all I could ever need is your open embrace – while you brush the fallen strands of hair out of my face – that by saying absolutely nothing your adoration is speaking volumes.

I know that there are times when I work too long; I think too much; I read too many journals and attend too many meetings and do too few dishes and laundry in return. But you have never once judged me for it. You have never once resented my commitment to what I do, because you understand that everything I give to my craft as a nurse I give to you ten fold. I think about you all of the time – the silliest notions remind me of you, but they do. I often brag about you to my patients and families, and they gush over photos and stories of our lives together. It is healing – for them and for me – to lead with distraction at times. And when I see the power of love in the form of wrinkled old skin and a tuft of white hair sitting quietly at the bedside, admiring the weakened other half as though they are foolish teenagers – I am reminded that everyone experiences love and loss: only few gain a lifetime. Thank you for being my lifetime.

To My (Future) Children:

I understand that I probably drive you crazy more often than not. It must be difficult to deal with a parent that plans for every worst-case scenario. What you do not realize is that I have lived through all kinds of worst-case scenarios, and I am not sure how I would bear being in those shoes. I know it must be silly that you only go to the doctor's office when you are really, really sick. It must be incredibly annoying that I sometimes make you wash your hands before AND after going to the bathroom. And I'm sure that you are irritated when I am the only parent missing from holidays, sporting events, and weekend activities. Just remember that while I am sleeping – day or night – I am resting up to care for other people and annoy them just as much as I annoy you! You didn't choose to have a parent that is a nurse, but I promise you, someday I believe that you will look to me as a valuable resource and, I hope, a wonderful parent. I may have moments when I am cranky and short with you, and I apologize for those times, but my days are very stressful and sometimes I may need just a few moments to recharge my batteries before continuing with my day. I work my hardest to provide you with more than just stuff – I hope to instill in you work ethic; compassion; curiosity; and a true passion for living every single day its fullest capacity. This may sound crazy today, but I hope that you someday look to others and say proudly, "My parent is a nurse!" I love you more than anything in this world, and thanks to what I do every day, I am constantly reminded to soak up every moment I have with you before you pursue your own dreams and ignite your own passions.

To My Parents:

I understand that you were at some point led to believe that the only two professions in this country are "doctor" or "lawyer." Since you have evolved and grown older, you have since recognized the true value in what my profession is and just how much I do. You have both instilled in me such a strong sense of integrity and discipline that I pray that this inner strength translates to the work that I do. I know that there are some misconceptions about what it takes to be a nurse; what they do daily; the extent of their autonomy; etcetera. However you have never once questioned my decision to become a nurse and utilize my critical thinking skills and academic pursuits in professional practice every single day. As you both grow older, I hope that my professional life can guide you into the lifestyle choices and health decisions that will leave you with the highest quality and quantity. I often judge my patients based on the two of you – I will think, "Man, he is dad's age!" or "She is younger than my mother!" What that means is this: I am thinking of you both even when I cannot come and see you. I can't deny that I often worry about you and how you are managing, but I have come to trust that if you truly have a concern you will always come to me with it. I am a nurse, but I am also your child. I will do anything in my power to provide you both with whatever physical, spiritual, or emotional companionship I can come to offer. Thank you for raising me to become a person who will advocate for the safety and security of others. Thank you for letting me share in your life experiences, allowing them to shape my own. Most of all, thank you for leading as examples that would make for all the trappings of a nurse.

To My Family and Friends

As you may have figured out, "Sorry, I'm working that day" is a running theme that you've come to encounter. It's not that I don't want to have lunch with you. It's not that I would rather be at the hospital than at your birthday. It's not that I am too lazy to make a schedule switch than to attend your barbecue. What it comes down to is this: when I became a nurse, I was obligated to the sacrifices that come with the role. Weekends and holidays at work are not simply endured by me alone – all of my colleagues must make choices that they sometimes do not prefer for the sake of our duties and obligations. We wish we could be there with you for every event that comes up; every phone call we've missed; and every group outing that arises – but that is simply not our reality. I thank you for continuing to reach out to me despite my often-busy schedule – there is no greater feeling than when we can connect and spend time with one another. I am so grateful for your camaraderie and for being there when I need you, despite having to listen to stories that might make you lose your lunch. I cannot tell you how much it means to me when we can sit together and laugh – truly laugh from the depths of our bellies and feel alive. Likewise, I cannot tell you how cleansing it is when we sit together in near silence and cry. What you confide in me, and many times, what I to you, are some of the deepest connections that we as human beings have to offer one another. Thank you for allowing me to remain myself while still evolving and growing. Your friendship is something that I always cherish, and while there will be weeks when I need nothing more than the sound of silence to center my balance, I will always hear you in my heart. Also, you should definitely have that rash looked at...

To My Patients

You have every reason to be angry with me. I may have been late with your pain medication. I might have forgotten an extra pillow. I likely asked your family to step out due to a situation that took place on the unit. But I assure you, if you only knew just how often I think about you, you would likely give me the benefit of the doubt. Because you see, in addition to ensuring that you are safe, stable, and comfortably taken care of, I am likely doing the same for others. What you might see as me taking my time to conduct a task is most likely due to some other priority that I had been forced to place above it. Whether you are a nurse with eight patients on a busy medical unit or you have one critically ill patient in intensive care, you are never truly free to focus on simply what is "yours." While your family complained that I did not feed you, they may have misunderstood that the procedure planned for you requires nothing to eat or drink. While you angrily yelled at the nursing assistant for waiting on a bedpan, I was assisting with a cardiac arrest on the other side of the floor. And while you were concerned with the hold up for your pain medications, I was frantically connecting with the pharmacy to ensure that your pills could be brought to me as soon as possible.

And yet, despite the fact that you sometimes become upset and frustrated and direct your emotions at me, I know one thing for certain: it is not truly me that concerns you. You are exhausted. You are frightened. You are in pain and you are poked and prodded and asked a million questions. Every day you meet a different person with a different title asked to treat a different body part. Or worse yet, you are intubated and sedated and require life-sustaining medications to pull you from the cold grasp of death. You are a human being who is dealing with the fragility of your own existence, and it is no wonder that I am your moving target. Despite all of this I want to make one thing perfectly clear: you are my priority. You are my baby. You are my largest project and greatest concern. I want you to understand that you may claim to hate me, but I will still help you. You may cause uproar, but I will still calm you. You may keep me busy, but I will still choose you: over eating, drinking, peeing, and sometimes leaving. As long as your heart is beating – and often when it is not – I will fight for you. And after a long day of honoring the beauty of life by saving yours; after an arduous night of embracing the end by helping you transition; after an exhausting shift of scratching tooth and nail to keep you with us, but losing you anyway: I hope you realize that I try my damndest to leave work at the door, but I cannot help but carry you with me.

Thank you for trusting me to care for you. Thank you for being the eternal "patient patient." Thank you for giving me a reason, every single day, to keep on fighting.

To My Physician and Advanced Practice Team

I understand that I can be a squeaky wheel sometimes, pushing a subject that was apparently addressed or had already resolved. It's simply that my patient or family has a request to see you, and despite my consolation, they are anxiously awaiting your insights. Thank you for your collaborative approach to caring for our patients, and for seeking my input on matters of patient care. I understand that you are busy and have a packed schedule, but those moments when you make the time to really address my issues are always remembered. I apologize for questioning your judgment at times – I simply see my patient for extended periods of time, and I believe that I can help you guide his or her care. I make no apologies, however, in advocating for those under my charge – what good would I be to this team if I did not fight for those who cannot? Although there are moments when we do not see eye-to-eye, I respect you and appreciate your practice. During those moments when you compliment my care to patients and their families, I truly feel like a colleague that can be trusted with even the most complicated situation. Those moments speak volumes of why I work as hard as I do, and they fuel the fire to consistently practice at the highest level of my craft...even when it means a 3:00am phone call for stool softener.

Thank you for the coffee. Thank you for the bagels. Thank you for working with me, side by side, in making a difference every day.

To My Fellow Nurses, I'm No Angel

I sit here staring at a blank computer screen, filled with quiet concern. It's simply that I have so many things to say to you, my many fellow nurses, and not enough time in the world to say it. You are my team. You are my posse. You are my family – an utterly dysfunctional one, but family at that. I believe that few professions exist where we can be grossly irritated by each other one moment, and cracking jokes in the next. It has been mentioned before that what we do every day makes us akin to the "Navy Seals" of the healthcare profession. That statement alone suggests we are working in some of the most stressful environments while enduring more intense circumstances daily than many face in a lifetime. What we do, every single day, is a labor of love. But we are all in on the real secret: nurses are not angels placed on earth to serve and lift. We are not diminutive and submissive and gentle souls that kiss boo-boos. We are not the starched white caps and perfectly polished shoes that history books portray. Nor are we fishnet stockings and naughty *rendezvous in dark corners. We have been glamorized and fetishized and placed on a pedestal unlike any other profession, and yet the definition of what we are is only surpassed by the list of what we are not.*

Our Dirty Little Secret

Many will never understand the extent of what we do every single shift. They can only imagine that it's a difficult profession (though they might never feel the weight of our feet, the ache in our backs, and the pain in our hearts at the end of it all). Some will say, "I wanted to be a nurse, but I could never do it." We smile and say something along the lines of, "Yup, it's a hard job but a good one," without a second thought, understanding that most people truly couldn't endure what we face every single day. Others might tell us how intelligent we are, and insist we attend medical school to become doctors. As much as we respect physicians, most of us don't want to become them. The connections we make and the difference we incite in our patients lives are worth the countless pitfalls and sacrifices we face.

None of them are in on our secret. Patients and families; husbands and wives; parents and children and colleagues and friends: because while they try, they will never understand the depth and breadth of mind and body required of a nurse. Some might question that statement – how hard could it really be? Isn't it only three shifts every week? Don't you earn overtime and receive bonuses every year? It's harder than they could ever imagine. It's more raw and real than they could ever dream. Yet when something truly incredible happens, and we get to be a part of it, nursing becomes a drug unlike any other.

What a miracle! Families will shout.

The work of modern medicine! Physicians will declare.

And yet those who are in on the secret, or at least are suspicious of it, understand that it was no miracle that saved your loved one. Rather, it was the intent and vigilant care of a critically thinking, intuitive, and fiercely devoted nurse. Our secret is that we save more lives than we are willing to admit; we catch more errors than we hope to share; and we can sense subtle nuances that prevent a turn for the worse. The nursing profession is oft touted as a humble one – a life of service to others through altruistic compassion. Yet here we are, with our dirty little secret: our filthy mouths; our dark humor and sarcastic sensibilities; snarky and sassy and smart – can you sense that? Oh no, we are not all nuns in nurses' clothing! We can be vicious. We can be vile. We can devour our young and destroy our reputations – we are not the perfect pictures you had envisioned – far from it.

We are Human

We are human. We make mistakes. We pick fights. We become emotional. And we must. Because every single day we grapple with our own identities, not only as men and women but also as nurses – defined by a role that we wear as a badge of honor, yet has the potential to become a Scarlet Letter. We are in a constant state of battle: with the establishment; with disease; with matters of life and death; with our colleagues and our families and ourselves. What we take on when we clock in every morning or evening is far more powerful than just a job – it is a struggle to give 99% of your being to others while never releasing that

164

final 1% of yourself. We are human. We are not infallible. We drink too much. We smoke too much. We eat candy bars for dinner. We take it out on you because there is nobody else to punch with our sack full of baggage. We are in one of the few businesses where an emergency is genuinely and truly an emergency – everything else is just details. And so while we apologize for our shortcomings; and we are sorry for our attitudes; and we hope to evolve into more compassionate and patient people everyday – we make no apologies about being nurses. Take us as we are, all of us – the beauty, the burdens – every ounce of us, because we did not choose to be this way. Somehow, even if you fight against it, becoming a nurse will find you. It will seep into the marrow of your bones. It will sink into your soul. You will sacrifice parts of your own being to protect perfect strangers, and it will feel like a totally rational thing to do.

It is not rational. It borders on crazy. We're all a touch too neurotic; a smidgen too type-A; a little too caring and bit too self-invested. I walked away from a 9-5 corporate career to pursue what was calling me. I ignored it, I fought it, but the nurse stirred from within and enveloped herself around me. And now? I will never be the same. I border on crazy. I'm slightly irrational. I'm absolutely neurotic. I'm completely invested. I'm a woman. I'm a wife. I'm a daughter. I'm a friend. But through it all – I am unapologetically a nurse.

You've come a long way, baby! Some day, you'll read this book back and smile: you once were a new nurse, and you've evolved into an unapologetic member of this deliciously confusing clan. My hope for you is that you walk through the doors of wherever it is you work, and allow yourself to experience the moment. Soak in everything – the highest of highs and the shit beneath your shoes lows – and allow it to simmer in your nursing arsenal. Whether you are new or feel the need to be renewed, I hope that you realize that others out there have survived your struggle. Others have fought your battle. Many have partaken in your plight. I understand that this book is only a fraction of the wisdom, stories, and guidance contained within the pinkie toe of many nurses out there, so allow me to provide merely your initial dip into the nursing pool. Explore your profession. Research your craft. And when the time comes that you've grown from being fresh and filled with fear into someone very different – don't forget to share your stories, and mine, with another nurse who just stepped into your shiny white shoes. Work hard. Laugh every day. Reflect on why you chose this life. And if you're going to be a nurse, remain unapologetically true to the man or woman beneath the scrubs. You are one of us now. Welcome to the family! Sending you alert and oriented wishes and PTO dreams!

Unapologetically yours,
A Former Newbie Nurse